A

TREATISE

ON

GYMNASTICKS,

TAKEN CHIEFLY FROM THE GERMAN OF

F. L. JAHN.

NORTHAMPTON, MASS.
PUBLISHED BY SIMEON BUTLER.....SOLD BY
HILLIARD, GRAY & CO. BOSTON....G. & C. CARVILL, NEW YORK....
CAREY, LEA, & CAREY, PHILADELPHIA....E. J. COALE, BALTIMORE....PISHEY THOMPSON, WASHINGTON.

T. WATSON SHEPARD, PRINTER.
1828.

DISTRICT OF MASSACHUSETTS...TO WIT:

DISTRICT CLERK'S OFFICE.

BE IT REMEMBERED, that on the sixth day of December, A. D. 1827, in the fifty-second year of the Independence of the United States of America, CHARLES BECK, of the said District, has deposited in this Office the title of a book, the right whereof he claims as Proprietor, in the words following, to wit:

"A Treatise on Gymnasticks, taken chiefly from the German of F. L. Jahn."

In conformity to the act of the Congress of the United States, entitled "An act for the encouragement of learning, by securing the copies of maps, charts and books, to the authors and proprietors of such copies, during the times therein mentioned:" and also an act, entitled, "An act supplementary to an act, entitled, An act for the encouragement of learning, by securing the copies of maps, charts and books to the authors and proprietors of such copies during the times therein mentioned; and extending the benefits thereof to the arts of designing, engraving and etching historical and other prints."

JOHN W. DAVIS, *Clerk of the District of Massachusetts.*

This scarce antiquarian book is included in our special *Legacy Reprint Series*. In the interest of creating a more extensive selection of rare historical book reprints, we have chosen to reproduce this title even though it may possibly have occasional imperfections such as missing and blurred pages, missing text, poor pictures, markings, dark backgrounds and other reproduction issues beyond our control. Because this work is culturally important, we have made it available as a part of our commitment to protecting, preserving and promoting the world's literature. Thank you for your understanding.

PREFACE.

In bringing before the public a work on a subject which has, of late, attracted deserved attention, I consider it proper to give a brief account of its origin, peculiarity, and use.

The same causes which occasioned the publication of the original, in Germany, about twelve years ago, render a translation desirable in this country. F. L. JAHN was the first in Germany who established a gymnasium on a scale, appropriated for the use of the community at large. Attempts of a more limited nature had been made before, but without ever extending beyond the bounds of their birth-place. It is, by no means, my intention to depreciate the value of these attempts; on the contrary, I believe that those who take an interest in the cause of physical education, would be pleased to become acquainted with the exertions of *Gutsmuths*, and several other men, years before *Jahn* came forward. Gymnasticks were known and practised in various places, but *Jahn* was the author of them as a national institution. How well he understood the deficiency of our education in this respect, and how successful he was in discovering and applying the remedies, is proved, beyond any reasonable doubt, by the establishment of gymnasiums, after his model, in almost every town of Germany, in the course of six or seven years. There is no exaggeration in asserting, that all the youth of Germany, and probably of many other countries, in a few years would have practised gymnasticks as an established part of regular education, had not several of the arbitrary governments of Germany at once put a stop to them, considering them, and rightly, a powerful engine of political freedom.

The applications made to *Jahn* from all parts of the country, for advice and information in establishing gymnasiums, and directing the exercises, were so frequent that they induced him to render his experience more accessible to the public by publishing a treatise on Gymnasticks, which has become the standard not only of most gymnasiums in Germany, but also in France and England.

The school of Messrs. COGSWELL & BANCROFT, in Northampton, Mass. was the first institution in this country, that introduced gymnastick exercises as a part of the regular instruction, in the spring of 1825. Since that time, the interest for this branch of education has been rapidly increasing, and frequent inquiries have been made respecting a subject much esteemed for its expected salutary effects, but little known as to its particulars. Besides this proof of the want of a work accessible to the consultations of every one, more distinct wishes were expressed to me, by several of the most zealous and able friends and advocates of physical education, to translate a work which would be suitable for this purpose, or compile one from the rich existing materials. Although I delayed, for a considerable time, entering upon the undertaking, in the hope that another, more able, might deliver me from the task, I did not doubt to which of the two ways proposed to give the preference. I fixed upon the treatise of *Jahn*, from reasons contained in the preceding lines.

My principal object in executing the translation, has been to exclude whatever is extraneous to a systematical illustration of gymnastick exercises, and to copy the accuracy and brevity of the original in describing the single exercises, as much as possible. There are several subjects closely connected with gymnasticks as a branch of education, highly interesting, which will present themselves to the mind of every reflecting examiner of Gymnasticks, and a few of which I will mention, with the wish that they might become the subjects of impartial and thorough investigation: The effect of the single exercises upon the constitution, and the particular members of the body.—The practical application of the single exercises for particular pursuits and occupations.—The advantages, derived by a republic from gymnastick exercises, uniting in one occupation all the different classes of the people, and thus forming a new tie for those who, for the most part, are widely separated by their different education and pursuits of life.—Of the connexion of instruction in gymnasticks with that of the other branches in institutions for educating instructers for their profession. However useful, and I would say necessary, a thorough examination of these and several other subjects might be, they have been excluded from this work as not strictly belonging to a system of gymnasticks.

As to the description of the exercises themselves, I was aware that a profusion of words, not only does not accomplish what is intended, to convey a clear and correct idea, but, on the contrary, occasions misunderstanding and confusion. Only the essential parts, and the distinguishing peculiarities of each exercise, ought to be enumerated in due succession, and I have endeavored to accomplish this end, by following closely the original which is really distinguished by the plastic power with which it describes the exercises.

This was by no means an easy task. The first difficulty lies in the thing itself, the subject being a new one. We are not accustomed to observe bodily movements with such accuracy, as to retain in our memory with ease, their single parts in their succession. Hence the difficulty for a writer to give, and for a reader to receive, a distinct idea of a given movement, through the medium of a description; and this will be the case, until, by general practice, we shall be enabled to discover the essential parts in every movement, whether we see it performed, or read a description of it.

Although I had a most excellent prototype in the original, yet the genius of both languages is so different, and the German of Jahn so peculiar that I could not make use of all which I found in the original. It is a well known fact that a subject, whether it be entirely new, or only more attended to, will exercise an influence upon the language, in proportion to its importance; it will either coin new words, or transplant them from other languages, or impart a new shade or greater distinctness of meaning to some already existing. This, I have no doubt, will be the case respecting gymnastick exercises, in however a limited extent, if the practice of them should be continued and propagated in this country and England. But, at present, there arises from this very circumstance, a difficulty which would have checked and fettered one whose vernacular tongue is the English, much more a foreigner, and one who has, but for a short time, been acquainted with the language of his adopted country. He is not the person calculated to make any of the changes mentioned; it would be presumption, to treat thus a language which is not his own; he would be subject to the grossest mistakes against the genius of the language.

I endeavored, through the whole work, to avoid this fault, though I frequently felt the want of a word—climbing with hands and feet, and with hands alone (klettern and klimmen)—or of an accurate distinction between synonymous words—leaping, jumping, bounding, springing. In one instance I allowed myself a liberty with the word *crouching* (see Preparatory Exercises, page 3, V; and Vaulting, page 22, II). In common use, it signifies the posture when a person lowers the upper part of his body, bending his knees and hips, so that the knees approach the breast. I have applied the same term to the posture, when a person, by means of a spring, draws up his knees to his breast, which is, in fact, the same posture, with this difference, that in the former, the body rests on the ground, in the latter is in the air.

I cannot leave this subject without expressing the wish, that one possessing an equally thorough knowledge of the language, and of gymnastick exercises, might give his attention to this subject. If he should succeed in removing the most obnoxious difficulties, according to a principle easily perceived and obeyed, much trouble and confusion would be saved in future.

This work, both the original and the translation, is intended to guide the practice of gymnastick exercises. No one, therefore, should expect to receive a correct idea of gymnasticks through this work, unless he joins practical exercises to the perusal of it. Gymnasticks are an art, and theory and practice should never be separated. The work is a systematical series of exercises, calculated to call forth the hidden, and to cultivate and increase the rude and infant strength; not a collection of single feats, which is a thing altogether foreign to our present object, and to Gymnasticks in general.

The original appeared without engravings or drawings, except those of the instruments. After Jahn had established his gymnasium in Berlin, the interest for gymnastick exercises was raised to such a height that, during the summer season, usually several individuals, from different parts of the country, spent some weeks or months in Berlin, to become familiarly acquainted with, and to propagate in their respective towns, gymnastick exercises. A treatise was necessary on a subject which spread so rapidly over the whole country, in order to direct, and prevent any extravagance or abuse of, the exercises; but drawings could be dispensed with, where the exercises were introduced into most places by those who had seen and exercised themselves. Not so here. The interest is neither so lively, nor the personal intercourse so easy, in a country of so great an extent. For this reason I resolved to aid the descriptions by a collection of engravings, drawn and engraved by Mr. Francis Graeter, a gentleman not only possessed of great skill in his art, but also familiarly acquainted with Gymnasticks. In order not to confound, rather than assist, and in order not to increase the expense to a degree, which would have rendered the work inaccessible to a large portion of the public, I confined myself, in each exercise to the fundamental, as it were, postures and movements.

Several important exercises are omitted, by no means from an idea that they may be neglected, but because they can be easily acquired, or are so extensive and complicated that a satisfactory treatment would exceed the limits of this treatise. To this description belong especially Fencing, Riding, Swimming, and military Exercises.

If the present work facilitates the introduction and management of gymnastick exercises, my wish is fulfilled, and I shall consider myself richly rewarded for the trouble which the execution of it occasioned.

CHARLES BECK.

Northampton, Mass. January, 1828.

CONTENTS.

FIRST SECTION.
GYMNASTICK EXERCISES.

I. PREPARATORY EXERCISES	1
Posture	1
1. Standing on tiptoe	2
II. Walking on tiptoe	2
III. Hopping	2
IV. Kicking	2
V. Crouching	3
VI. Hopping on one foot	4
VII. Straddling	5
VIII. Raising of one thigh	5
IX. Crossing	6
X. Stretching	6
II. WALKING	7
I. Grace	7
II. Duration	8
III. Quickness	8
IV. Indifference as to locality	8
III. RUNNING	8
Instruments	8
a. Raceground	8
b. Circles	8
Posture	9
Precautions	9
Different modes of running	9
A. *Running straight*	9
I. Racing	9
II. Running with a view to duration	9
B. *Running in the circle*	10
I. Racing	10
II. Running with a view to duration	10
C. *Running in straight lines and angles*	10
Running in a spiral line	10
Another kind of running	11
Running backwards	11
Running up a hill	11

IV. LEAPING 11
 Preparatory exercises . . . 11
 Of leaps in general . . . 11
  I. Leap from the spot . . . 12
  II. Leap with a preparatory spring . . 12
  III. Leap with running . . . 12
  Two particular kinds of leaping . . 12
 A. Free Leaping 13
  1. Long Leap 13
   a. forwards 13
   b. sideways 13
   c. oblique 13
   d. turning 14
   e. backwards 14
  Leaping in large numbers . . 14
  2. High Leap 14
   Instrument 14
   Variations of the Leap . . 14
   Degrees of height . . . 15
   Leaping in large numbers . . 15
  Long and high Leap . . . 15
  3. Deep Leap 16
   Instrument 16
  Deep and long Leap . . . 16
 B. Leaping with a pole . . . 16
  Instruments 16
   Leaping-stand . . . 16
   Leaping-poles . . . 16
   Holding of the pole . . . 17
  I. Long Leap 17
  II. High Leap 18
   Long and high leap . . . 18
  III. Deep Leap 18
   Deep and long leap . . . 18
   Leap with two poles . . . 18

V. VAULTING 19
 Instruments 19
  Vaulting-bar 19
  Vaulting-horse 20
 Preparatory exercises . . . 21
  I. Hopping 21
  II. Crouching 22
  III. Straddling 22
  IV. Raising one leg . . . 22
  V. Crossing 22
  VI. Pushing off 22
  VII. Raising 22

VIII.	Swinging	23
IX.	Swinging with raising the knees	23
X.	Moving along, resting upon the hands	23
	Rules to be observed in Vaulting	23

A. *Simple Vaults* 25
  a. Vaults from the side . . 25
    I. First mounting and alighting . . 25
    II. Second mounting and alighting . 26
    III. Third vault and alighting . . 26
    IV. Fourth vault . . . 27
    V. Fifth vault . . . 27
    VI. Sixth vault . . . 27
    VII. Seventh vault . . . 28
    VIII. Eighth vault . . . 28
    IX. Ninth vault . . . 28
    X. Tenth vault . . . 28
    XI. Eleventh vault . . . 28
  b. Vaults from behind . . 29
    I. First vault . . . 29
    II. Second vault . . . 30
    III. Third vault . . . 30
    IV. Fourth vault . . . 31
    V. Fifth vault . . . 31
    VI. Sixth vault and alighting . . 31
      a. by hopping off . . 32
      b. by another vault . . 32
    VII. Seventh vault . . . 32
    VIII. Eighth vault . . . 32
    IX. Ninth vault . . . 32
    X. Tenth vault . . . 33
    XI. Eleventh vault . . . 33
      a. forwards . . 34
      b. backwards . . 34
    Alighting . . . 34
  Some more simple vaults . . 34
    I. Mounting . . . 35
    II Second vault . . . 35
    III. Third vault . . . 35
    IV. Fourth vault . . . 35
    V. Fifth vault . . . 35
    VI. Sixth vault . . . 35
    VII. Seventh vault . . . 36
    VIII. Eighth vault . . . 36
  Fencing vaults, or vaults with one hand . 37
    I. Mounting . . . 37
    II. Third vault from the side . . 37
    III. Fourth vault from the side . . 37

IV. Fifth vault from the side	37
V. Fifth vault, between the fourth and eighth vaults from the side	37
VI. Sixth vault from behind	37
VII. Eighth vault from behind	38
VIII. Eleventh vault from behind	38
B. *Compound Vaults*	38
I. First vault	38
II. Second vault	38
III. Third vault	39
IV. Fourth vault	39
V. Fifth vault	40
VI. Sixth vault	40
VII. Seventh vault	40
VIII. Eighth vault	41
IX. Ninth vault	41
X. Tenth vault	41
XI. Eleventh vault	41
XII. Twelfth vault	42
C. *Continued Vaults*	42
I. Fourth vault from the side	42
II. Fifth " " "	43
III. Eighth " " "	44
IV. Eleventh " " "	45
D. *Double Vaults*	45
I. First and Second Mounting	45
II. Third vault from the side	45
III. Fourth " " "	45
IV. Fifth " " "	45
V. Eighth " " "	45
VI. Third vault from the side, and sixth vault from behind	45
VII. Third vault from the side, and first vault from behind	46
VIII. Sixth vault from behind	46
IX. First " " "	46
E. *Threefold Vaults*	46
I. Eighth vault from the side	46
II. Third and eighth vaults from the side	46
III. Fourth and eighth vaults from the side	46
IV. Sixth and eighth vaults from behind	46
F. *Free Vaults*	47
I. High leap	47
II. Eleventh vault from behind	47
a. Exercises with the head foremost	47
I. Eleventh vault from behind	47
II. Eighth vault from the side	48

III. Third Exercise	48
IV. Fourth Exercise	48
V. Fifth Exercise	48
b. Exercises in a suspended position	48
I. First Exercise	48
II. Second Exercise	48
Leap-frog	48
VI. BALANCING	49
Instruments	49
1. Lying bar	49
2. Suspended bar	49
3. Small bar	49
4. Post	49
5. Plank	50
6. Board	50
Preparatory Exercises	50
I. Standing on one leg	50
II. Walking on the juncture of two boards	50
III. Walking with legs stretched far, and raised high	50
Exercises	50
I. Balancing walk	50
II. Passing by one another	50
III. Taking up something	51
IV. Sitting down	51
V. Fifth Exercise	51
VI. Raising one foot	51
VII. Balancing combat	51
A. *Walking on Stilts*	51
Instruments	51
Holding of the stilts	52
I. Walking	52
II. Running	52
III. Hopping on one stilt	52
IV. Ascending and descending steps	52
B. *Scating*	53
Instruments	53
Mode of fastening	53
Preparatory Exercises	54
I. Standing on scates	54
II. Gliding	54
Variations of scating	54
I. Scating in straight lines	54
II. Scating in circular lines	55
a. outwards	55
b. inwards	56
III. Some other kinds of scating	56

   a. Scating in a serpentine line . 56
   b. Scating in a straight line towards the side 56
   c. Scating in a circular line, described by
    both feet 57
   d. Scating with stepping over . 57
VII. EXERCISES ON THE SINGLE BAR . . 57
  Instruments 57
   1. Single bar . . . 57
   2. Sliding bar . . . 58
 Explanations 58
  I. Hanging 58
   a. Side-hanging . . . 58
   b. Cross-hanging . . . 58
  II. Grasp 58
   a. in side-hanging . . 58
    1. from above . . . 58
    2. from beneath . . . 58
    3. double grasp . . . 58
   b. in cross-hanging . . 58
  III. Situation upon the bar . . 58
   a. Sitting 58
    1. Side-seat . . . 58
    2. Riding-seat . . . 58
   b. Resting . . . 59
   c. Being suspended . . 59
    1. from the position of sitting . 59
    2. from the position of resting 59
A. *Exercises in Hanging* . . . 59
  I. Hanging on . . . 59
  II. Hanging close to the bar . . 60
  III. Hanging in a suspended position . 62
  IV. Hanging down . . . 62
  V. Moving in Hanging . . 63
   Instrument 63
  VI. Raising the body . . . 64
  VII. Changing the grasp . . 65
  VIII. Transition from the position of hanging on
   to the position of resting on the bar 66
  IX. Moving the body, resting on, or suspended
   by, the arms . . . 66
  X. Lowering and Raising . . 67
B. *Exercises with Swinging* . . . 67
 Preparatory Exercises . . . 67
  I. Sitting 67
  II. Changing the seat . . 68
 Exercises 69
  I. Swinging up . . . 70
   First kind 70

CONTENTS.

Second kind	71
Third kind	71
Fourth kind	72
Fifth kind	73
II. Swinging around	73
a. First kind	73
b. Second kind	75
c. Third kind	75
d. Fourth kind	76
e. Fifth kind	76
f. Sixth kind	76
III. Swinging off	76
a. with an entire revolution	76
b. with half a revolution	77
IV. Swinging through	78
V. Swinging under	79
VI. Swinging forwards and backwards	79
Series of exercises for practice	79
VIII. EXERCISES ON THE PARALLEL BARS	83
Instrument	83
A. *Exercises with Raising, Resting, and Bearing up*	84
I. Hopping	84
II. Lowering and rising	85
III. Lowering and touching the bars	85
IV. Lowering upon the elbows and rising	85
V. Raising	86
VI. Suspending	86
VII. Passing over the bar	86
a. forwards	86
b. backwards	87
VIII. Moving along upon the hands	87
IX. Turning	88
B. *Exercises with Swinging*	88
I. Changing the seat	88
II. Swinging over the bar before the arms	89
III. Swinging over the bar, behind the arms	90
IV. Changing the seat from one bar over the other, before the hands, with alighting	90
V. Changing the seat from one bar over the other, behind the hands, with alighting	91
VI. Changing the seat, on the same bar, with alighting	91
VII. Changing the seat from one bar, before the hands, to the other, behind the hands, with alighting	92
VIII. Eighth exercise	93
IX. Circle	93
X. Swinging	94

CONTENTS.

XI. A combination of lowering upon the elbows, and rising, with swinging	96
XII. A combination of moving along, upon the hands, with swinging	96
XIII. Swinging off	96
XIV. Turning over	97
Pushing through	97
IX. CLIMBING	97
Instruments	97
1. Climbing-pole	97
2. Climbing-mast	97
3. Climbing-rope	98
4. Ladders	98
a. wooden ladder	98
b. rope-ladder	98
5. Slant or oblique poles and masts	98
Arrangements of the instruments	98
1. Single mast	98
2. Climbing-stand of two masts	99
3. Climbing-stand of four masts	99
4. Instrument for climbing by means of the arms alone	99
A. *Climbing, properly so called*	100
Directions for Climbing	100
I. Climbing on the pole	101
II. Climbing on the mast	101
III. Climbing on the slant pole	101
IV. Climbing on the rope	101
V. Climbing on the ladder	102
B. *Climbing by means of the arms alone*	103
I. with a grasp when the plane of the hand is perpendicular	103
II. with a grasp when the plane of the hand is horizontal	103
X. THROWING	104
A. *Shooting*	105
𝕬. *with fire-arms*	105
Instruments	105
a. Rifle	105
b. Aim	105
Charging	106
Posture	107
Aiming	107
Preparatory Exercises	107
I. Shot in a perpendicular line	107
II. Shot in a horizontal line	107
III. Combination of the two preceding exercises	107

Exercises	108
Precautions	109
B. with the cross-bow	109
C. with the bow	109
Instruments	109
a. bow	109
b. arrow	110
Holding the bow	110
D. with the dart	110
Instruments	110
a. dart	110
b. aim	111
Position	111
Preparatory Exercises	112
Exercises	112
I. Throw in a straight line	112
II. Throw in a curved line	112
III. Throw in a declining line	113
B. Throwing by means of swinging the arm stretched forwards and backwards	113
Instrument	113
Place	113
Aim	114
Position	114
Method of throwing	114
Throwing with a discus	114
C. Throwing by stretching the arm which was before bent	115
Place	115
Instrument	115
Mode of throwing	115
Position	115
Exercise in pushing	115
D. Throwing an iron bar	116
Instrument	116
Posture	116
Mode of throwing	116
E. Slinging	116
I. Slinging by means of the hands alone, or common throwing	116
II. Slinging by means of particular instruments	117
F. Ricocheter	117
G. Throwing ducks and drakes	117
XI. DRAWING	117
Instruments	117
1 Rope	117
2. Instrument for drawing with the neck	117

CONTENTS.

3 Staves	117
A. *Drawing with the hands*	117
I. with the hands alone	117
II. by means of instruments	118
a. on the rope	118
b. on the rope, passing over a roller	118
c. on the staff	118
Raising a person	118
B. *Drawing with the neck*	119
a. standing	119
b. resting on hands and feet	119
XII. PUSHING	119
A. Pushing of an adversary	119
B. Pushing on a particular instrument	120
Instrument	120
XIII. LIFTING	120
I. Lifting an instrument to measure the strength of the arms	120
a. a staff	120
b. a box	120
II. Lifting a balance-beam	121
III Holding of sand-bags or weights	121
XIV. CARRYING	121
A. Carrying inanimate bodies	122
I. with the hands	122
II. on the shoulders	122
B. Carrying a man	122
I. on the back	122
II. on the shoulders	122
III. on the hands	122
XV. EXERCISES WITH DUMB-BELLS	123
Instrument	123
Preparatory Exercises	123
Posture	123
Exercises	124
XVI. WRESTLING	125
Place	125
Position	125
Grasp	125
Preparatory Exercises	126
Exercises	126
XVII. SKIPPING WITH THE HOOP	128
Instrument	128
Exercises	128
XVIII. SKIPPING WITH THE ROPE	129
A. *with the short rope*	129
Instrument	129

Carriage	129
I. Simple Skipping	129
II. Double Skipping	130
III. Turning	130
B. *with the long rope*	130
Instrument	130
Exercises	131
Appendix	132
A number of single exercises	132

SECOND SECTION.

GYMNASTICK GAMES.

Of Gymnastick Games in general	141
Description of some games	142
A. Games which may be played in the gymnasium itself	142
B. Games which are to be played without the precincts of the gymnasium	144

THIRD SECTION.

MANAGEMENT OF A GYMNASIUM.

Management of a gymnasium	151
I. Of the instructor in gymnasticks	152
II. Of the exercises	153
III. Of the time for exercises	155
IV. Of the dress	156
V. Of the resting-place	157
VI. Of the spectators	157
VII. Of the laws	157
A. General laws	158
B. Special laws	159
a. for running	159
b. for leaping	159
c. for vaulting	159
d. for balancing	160
e. for the single bar	160
f. for the parallel bars	160
g. for climbing	160
h. for throwing with lances	161
i. for throwing with balls	161
j. for wrestling	161
k. for games	161

FOURTH SECTION.

OF THE FOUNDATION AND ARRANGEMENT OF A GYMNASIUM.

I. Of the situation of a gymnasium	165
II. Of the shape of a gymnasium	166
III. Of the size of a gymnasium	168
IV. Of the apparatus of a gymnasium	169
Apparatus of a gymnasium for 400 pupils	170
Necessary apparatus for 80 pupils	172
V. Estimate of the apparatus of a gymnasium for 400 pupils	173

EXPLANATION OF THE PLATES.

PLATE I.

Fig. 1. Kicking or striking the breech with the heels, in apparent running. See Preparatory Exercises IV, b, page 3.

Fig. 2. Double striking. See Preparatory Exercises IV, c, page 3.

Fig. 3. Crouching with sitting. See Preparatory Exercises V, a, page 3.

Fig. 4. Crouching in leaping. See Preparatory Exercises V, b, page 4.

Fig. 5. Hopping on one foot. See Preparatory Exercises VI, page 4.

Fig. 6. Hopping on one foot through an arch, formed by taking hold of the raised foot with the opposite hand. See Preparatory Exercises VI, e, page 4.

Fig. 7. Raising of one thigh forwards. See Preparatory Exercises VIII, a, page 5.

Fig. 8. Raising of one thigh sideways. See Preparatory Exercises VIII, b, page 5.

Fig. 9. Raising of one thigh backwards. See Preparatory Exercises VIII, c, page 5.

Fig. 10. Crossing. See Preparatory Exercises IX, page 6.

Fig. 11. Stretching. See Preparatory Exercises X, page 6.

Fig. 12. Posture of the gymnick standing at the horse. See Vaulting, preparatory exercises, page 21.

Fig. 13. Hopping. See Vaulting, preparatory exercises I, page 21.

PLATE II.

Fig. 1. High leap without a pole. See Leaping, page 14.

Fig. 2. Holding of the pole. See Leaping, page 17.

Fig. 3. Posture of the gymnick resting on his arms upon the parallel bars. See page 84.

Fig. 4. Posture of the gymnick standing at the parallel bars. See page 84.

Fig. 5. Posture of the gymnick on the parallel bars, raising his legs forwards. See page 86, V.

Fig. 6. The gymnick in a suspended position on the parallel bars. See page 86, VI.
Fig. 7. Swinging on the parallel bars. See page 94, X.
Fig. 8. Climbing on the rope. See page 101, IV.
Fig. 9. Climbing on the pole. See page 101, I.
Fig. 10. Climbing on the mast. See page 101, II.

PLATE III.

Fig. 1. Crouching. See Vaulting, preparatory exercises II, page 22.
Fig. 2. Straddling. See Vaulting, preparatory exercises III, page 22.
Fig. 3. Pushing off. See Vaulting, preparatory exercises VI, page 22.
Fig. 4. Raising. See Vaulting, preparatory exercises VII, page 22.
Fig. 5. Swinging. See Vaulting, preparatory exercises VIII, page 23.
Fig. 6 Swinging with raising the knees. See Vaulting, preparatory exercises IX, page 23.
Fig. 7. Moving along, resting upon the hands. See Vaulting, preparatory exercises X, page 23.
Fig. 8. Posture of the gymnick sitting on the horse. See Vaulting, rules to be observed 5, page 24.

PLATE IV.

Fig. 1. Sitting upon the single bar, upon both thighs, see page 58.
Fig. 2. Sitting upon the single bar, upon one thigh, see page 59.
Fig. 3. Resting upon the single bar, see page 59.
Fig. 4. Being suspended, in the position of sitting, on the single bar, see page 59.
Fig. 5. Hanging down from the single bar, on the feet, see page 63, IV, a.
Fig. 6. Hanging down from the single bar, on the knees, see page 63, IV, b, 1.
Fig. 7. Hanging down from the single bar, on the toes, see page 63, IV, b, 2.
Fig. 8. Hanging down from the single bar, on the heels, see page 63, IV, b, 3.
Fig. 9. Hanging close to the bar from the position of cross-hanging, see page 60, II, a, 1.
Fig. 10. Hanging close to the bar from the position of side-hanging, see page 61, II, a, 2.
Fig. 11. Hanging in a suspended position, see page 62, III, a, 1.

EXPLANATION OF THE PLATES.   xxi

PLATE. V.

Fig. 1. Cross-hanging with the hands on the single bar, see page 59, A, I, a, 1.
Fig. 2. Cross-hanging with the arms, on the single bar, see page 59, A, I, a, 1.
Fig. 3. Side-hanging with the hands, grasping from above, on the single bar, see page 59, A, I, a, 2, а.
Fig. 4. Side-hanging with the lower part of the arms, grasping from above, on the single bar, see page 60, A, I, a, 2, а.
Fig. 5. Side-hanging with the upper part of the arms, grasping from above, on the single bar, see page 60, A, I, a, 2, а.
Fig. 6. Side-hanging with the hands, grasping from beneath, on the single bar, see page 60, A, I, a, 2, b.
Fig. 7. Side-hanging with the hands, double grasp, on the single bar, see page 60, A, I, a, 2, c.
Fig 8. Side-hanging, with the hands, behind the body, grasping from above, on the single bar, see page 60, A, I, b, 1.
Fig. 9. Side-hanging, with the lower part of the arms, behind the body, grasping from above, on the single bar, see page 60, A, I, b, 1.
Fig. 10. Side-hanging, with the hands, behind the body, grasping from beneath, on the single bar, see page 60, A, b, 2.
Fig. 11. Side-hanging, with the hands behind the body, grasping from either side, on the single bar, see page 60, A, b, 3.

PLATE VI.

Fig. 1. Throwing with a dart in a straight line, see page 112, I.
Fig. 2. Throwing with a dart in a curved line, see page 112, II.
Fig. 3. Throwing by means of swinging the arm stretched forwards and backwards, see page 114.
Fig. 4. Throwing by stretching the arm which was before bent, see page 115.
Fig. 5. Position for wrestling, see page 125.
Fig. 6. Wrestling with the entire grasp, see page 125.
Fig. 7. Wrestling with the half grasp, see page 125.
Fig. 8. Holding down, see Wrestling, page 126, V, a.
Fig. 9. Holding down, see Wrestling, page 126, V, b.
Fig. 10. Holding the hoop, see Skipping, page 128.
Fig. 11. Holding the rope, see Skipping, page 129.

PLATE. VII.

Fig. A. Leaping-stand. See Leaping, page 14 and 16.
Pig. B. Aim for throwing with a dart. See Throwing, page 111.

Fig. C. Dart. See Throwing, page 110.
Fig. D. Vaulting-bar. See Vaulting, page 19.
Fig. E, F, and G. Vaulting-horse. See Vaulting, page 20.
Fig. H, and I. Parallel bars. See page 83.
Fig. K and L. Single bar. See page 57.
Fig. M. Instrument for moving in hanging, see page 63.
Fig. N. Balancing-pole. See Balancing, page 49, 2.
Fig. O. Instrument for drawing. See Drawing, page 117, 2.

Plan of a gymnasium.

Fig. 1. Place 10 feet broad, for fences, hedges, and trees. See page 167.

Fig. 2. Entry 15 feet wide. See page 167.

Fig. 3. Walks or communications, some 5, some 10 feet wide. See page 167.

Fig. 4. Race-ground 400 feet long, 30 feet broad.
 a. Place of starting,
 b. Goal.
See Running, page 8.

Fig. 5. Circles in a place 70 feet long, 30 feet broad. See Running, page 8.

Fig. 6. Place 80 feet long, 40 feet broad, for
 a. Stands for leaping with poles, see Leaping, page 16,
 b. Stands for leaping without poles, see Leaping, page 14.

Fig. 7. Place 90 feet long, 40 feet broad, for
 a. a large ditch, see Leaping, page 17;
 b. a small ditch, see Leaping, page 13;
 c. steps, see Leaping, page 16.

Fig. 8. Place 240 feet long, 40 feet broad, for
 a. Vaulting-bars, without saddle-holds,
 b. Vaulting-bars, with saddle-holds, see Vaulting, page 19.

Fig. 9. Place 60 feet long, 30 feet broad, for
 a. a large balancing-bar,
 b. a small balancing-bar,
 c. a lying bar, see Balancing, page 49.

Fig. 10. Place 200 feet long, 30 feet broad, for single bars, see page 57.

Fig. 11. Place 120 feet long, 30 feet broad, for parallel bars, see page 83.

Fig. 12. Place 135 feet long, 40 feet broad, for
 a. Climbing-masts, see page 97;
 b. Climbing-stand of two masts, see page 99;
 c. Single mast, see page 98;
 d. Climbing-stand of four masts, see page 99;
 e. Instrument for climbing by means of the arms alone, see page 99;
 f. Instrument for Moving in hanging, see page 63.

EXPLANATION OF THE PLATES. xxiii

Fig. 13. Place 230 feet long, 40 feet broad, for
    a. Throwing with darts, see page 111;
    b. Drawing, see page 117.
Fig. 14. Place for Throwing with balls, first kind, 130 feet long, 60 feet broad; see page 114.
    a. Aim,
    b. Mound,
    c. Low mound.
Fig. 15. Place for Throwing with balls, second kind, 40 feet long, 30 feet broad, see page 115.
    a. Standing-place.
    b. Mound.
Fig. 16. Place 60 feet long, 60 feet broad, for
    a. the exercises with the long rope, see page 130;
    b. the exercises with the short rope, see page 129.
Fig. 17. Place for Wrestling, 60 feet square, see page 125.
Fig. 18. Place for Preparatory Exercises, 60 feet long, 40 feet broad, see page 1.
Fig. 19. Place for Playing 120 feet square; see page 142.
    a. the goals.
Fig 20. Place 150 feet long, 50 feet broad, see page 167.
    a. Place for rest.
    O. Place for publications.
    b. Building.
    c. Place for clothes.

PLATE VIII.

Fig. R. Single mast, see page 96.
Fig. S. Climbing-stand of two masts, see page 99.
Fig. T. Climbing-stand of four masts, see page 99.
Fig. V. Instrument for climbing by means of the arms alone, see page 99.
Fig. W and Z. Cross to be fixed on the top of the climbing-mast, see page 97.

1

FIRST SECTION.

GYMNASTICK EXERCISES.

I. PREPARATORY EXERCISES.

ALL preparatory exercises have for their object to strengthen and to render limber the lower extremities, and to accustom the body to a good carriage in general, as well as in single exercises. They cannot be sufficiently recommended, not only on account of their being preparatory to several other exercises, especially leaping and vaulting, but also on account of their being exceedingly useful in forming and strengthening the body. All instruction in gymnastick exercises ought to begin with them, and every individual to have acquired some facility and duration in performing them, before he passes over to other exercises. They are the more valuable, because they can be practised without any instruments, and by a large number at a time.

Posture:

Feet and knees must always be as close as possible.

Body erect, belly inwards, breast outwards. Particular care must be taken to maintain the posture of the upper part of the body. In this way alone the back can be drawn in, the shoulders recede, and a firm and noble posture of the body be effected.

Hands flat upon the hips, the thumb backwards, the fingers forward. Keeping the hands so prevents an unsteady wavering motion of the body.

Lips close.

I. *Standing on tiptoe* or, to speak more correctly, on the forepart of the foot. The gymnick raises the heels from the ground, and stands firmly on the forepart of the feet. The joints of the toes are strongly bent, and the knees stretched. This is to be practised for some time.

II. *Walking on tiptoe.* The knees must not bend, and the joints of the feet are to be extended considerably. The gymnick moves

    forwards,
    backwards,
    laterally, to the right and left side.

III. *Hopping.* The starting of the body from the ground in the posture on tiptoe.

  a. With the knees stiff; the body is raised by the elastic motion of the joints of the toes.

  b. With bending the knees; the knees bend a little, but are stretched, as soon as the toes have left the ground. At coming down upon the ground, the knees bend but a little.

Both these kinds of hopping are to be practised

  a. on the spot,
  b. moving from the place
    forwards,
    backwards,
    laterally to the right and left.

IV. *Kicking*, striking the breech with the heels. This motion exercises the flexibility of the knees still more than hopping with bending the knees. (III, *b.*).

  a. In running, forwards, backwards and laterally. While one foot touches the ground, the other strikes the breech, the right foot the right side, and the left, the left. The running must be slow, but the start from the ground high and in quick succession.

b. In apparent running. The preceding exercise, except that the gymnick remains on the spot. See pl. I, fig. 1.

c. Double striking. Both feet at a time strike the breech. The higher and easier the start, the better the exercise. This is one of the most important preparatory exercises.

    1. On the spot. See pl. I, fig. 2.

    2. Moving from the place, but with short jumps and good carriage of the body, forward, backward and laterally.

Practice will enable a man to repeat this exercise a hundred times without stopping.

d. Standing on both feet. While one foot strikes the breech, the other rests on the ground, either on the whole sole or, what is more difficult, on tiptoe.

e. Standing on one leg ; the other leg is stretched forwards, before it strikes against the breech.

f. Standing upon one foot and striking the breech with it; the most difficult kind of kicking. This exercise repeated twenty times in succession, produces great fatigue.

V. *Crouching* ; the contracted posture of the body, the knees approaching the breast.

    a. With sitting. The upper part of the body is perpendicular, the thighs horizontal, and the heels close to the breech.

    1. On the spot. See pl. I, fig. 3.

    2. Moving from the place
        forwards,
        backwards,
        laterally, to the right and left.

This exercise is very fatiguing on account of the strong bend of the knees ; but at the same time, it very much increases their flexibility.

practised over any suitable object, as a chair. The upper part of the body must not be influenced in its position by the movement of the leg. The resting leg must stand firmly. This kind occurs frequently in vaulting.

IX. *Crossing* is straddling with a spring, and crossing the legs alternately in descending. The more the gymnick separates the legs, and crosses without losing the balance, the better. See pl. I, fig. 10.

X. *Stretching*, when the body, from head to heels, forms a straight line. The different exercises of this kind consist either in preserving that position, or in moving in it, wherein the hands either assist, or rest close to the body. All of them are extremely strengthening to the joints of the back.

a. Stretching with the assistance of the hands. Rising on tiptoe, crouching, hands extended forwards, falling forwards of the body without touching the ground with the knees, stretching of the body, so that it does not bend, but forms a straight line. The arms are in a right angle with the body. To stretch them out in a larger angle, tires too soon. Remaining for some time in this posture. See pl. I, fig. 11.

Circling:

1. With the hands. The gymnick turns in the posture described above, so that the hands describe a circle, the feet forming the centre. The motion is first made to the right, then to the left. Great care must be taken not to sink or raise the back.

2. With the feet. The hands are in the centre, and the feet describe the circumference.

This circling can be performed:

1. the face towards the ground, and the feet resting upon the toes, or

2. the back towards the ground, and the feet resting on the heels. The latter is very difficult, but very exercising.

b. Stretching without the assistance of the hands. The hands are kept close to the body.

 1. To be raised from the ground by another person in a straight and stretched posture.

 2. To rest in a stretched posture over an excavation. This may be practised with three chairs, the middle one being taken away by the person himself: or upon a narrow joist resting on two chairs, with or without a balancing-pole.

 3. To stretch out one's self, when the legs, up to the knees, are held by another person on a bench or chair; the body is bent at the hips, so as to form a right angle, the knees being stretched at the same time.

II. WALKING.

A good walker must connect grace with quickness and perseverance, whatever be the nature of the ground, whether hilly, sandy, or slippery. To walk well, is a great art, and deserves to be attended to by parents from the earliest years of their children; for habit here, as in most cases, is all powerful. It is an exercise which may be practiced in any place, though not so well in a common exercise-ground as elsewhere.

1. *Grace.*

A straight natural carriage of the whole body, particularly of the head, without any thing artificial, or affected; a light, yet firm step with the whole sole of the foot at once; the knees straightened, whenever the foot touches the ground. The feet should be turned a little outwards.

The arms may move somewhat, but must not shake; the motion is to be made more with the lower, than the upper arm. The walk must not be crawling, jumping, waddling, nor staggering, it must be straight forward, and firm; the knees and ankles must not touch each other. The length of the steps must be in proportion to the size of the body, particularly of the lower limbs, so that the body may not lose its balance.

II. *Duration*, cannot be acquired except by much practice. Walks daily taken, and gradually increased, and then longer excursions and journies on foot, are requisite. Perseverance in walking and strength to carry some weight, is an important accomplishment. The knapsack, fastened with *two* straps on the shoulders, is always to be carried on the back.

III. *Quickness* of walking depends partly upon the length, partly on the quick repetition of the steps. Short and short-legged persons, therefore, should make up by the quickness of their steps what they want in length. It is a good exercise, to walk the same distance in a fixed and gradually shortened time.

IV. *Indifference as to locality.* Walking over unlevelled ground is much more difficult, but at the same time a greater exercise. The same is the case in walking through deep sand.

If a hill is so steep, that every step requires considerable exertion, then the motion is called *ascending*, which may be practised with and without a load.

III. RUNNING.

Running, if practised with precaution, is an exercise extremely salutary to the chest and lungs.

Instruments:

a. *Race-ground;* if possible, straight. It must not be overgrown with grass, nor covered with light sand, nor consist of clay which is soon made slippery by rain.

The width is 25 feet; the length any part of a mile; if possible, not under 200 feet. The beginning and end must be marked by signs fixed and easily seen. See pl. VII, fig. 4.

b. *Circles.* Three circles are described in a turfy ground, the centres of which lie in one straight line. The width of the path 18 inches; the diameter of each circle 20 feet. See pl. VII, fig. 5.

Posture of the body :

Breast out, shoulders back, upper part of the body forwards; upper arms close to the body, elbows bent, and kept backwards. The steps light, and with the ball of the foot, not with the whole sole. The mouth shut; breathing long, uniform, and more through the nose, than through the mouth.

Precautions.

Duration must be acquired by degrees, not attempted at first.

Cool and calm days are best for this exercise.

In the beginning run with, not against, the wind.

When very much heated, or out of breath, stop.

After running, cool yourself by walking about, not by standing still, nor lying down.

DIFFERENT MODES OF RUNNING.

A. Straight on without turning.
B. In the line of a circle.
C. In straight lines and angles.

These three modes may be practised in the manner of a *race*, or in *trotting*.

Measuring by estimation is to be practised, in order to find, whether a certain object may be reached by a quick or a slower pace.

A. RUNNING STRAIGHT.

I. *A race* may be performed on the race-ground by parties from six to eight; on a wider field by more. In the former case, if the comparative swiftness of the several numbers is to be tested, the time must be shewn by a chronometer.

II. *Running with a view to duration,* is to be practised on the race-ground. In racing, he gains the prize, who runs through the largest space in the shortest time, with the least exhaustion; in running with a view to duration, he, who runs through the largest space with the least exhaustion; in case of equality in these two respects, length of time, of course, decides.

B. RUNNING IN THE CIRCLE.

I. *Racing in the circle*, is to be practised in the place prepared for this purpose. See pl. VII, fig. 5. The arms and hands may assist in this kind of running by preserving the equilibrium. The party should consist of six. The runners stand in the first circle, at a distance of three or four paces from one another, and start at once; they run so, that they cross in a meandering manner, where two circles meet. He that is able to reach the person running before, strikes him slightly with the hand, and he who is struck, must leave the circle; likewise he who steps over the edge of the circle. He who remains last, is conqueror. The striking does not begin, until the runners have passed into the second circle.

II. *Running in the circle with a view to duration*, is to be performed in the same place. Number of circuits, length of time, and degree of exhaustion are to be computed. If several are running, they must keep equal steps and distance, in order to avoid disturbance.

C. RUNNING IN STRAIGHT LINES AND ANGLES.

It is of great use to make sudden short turns in running. This may be practised about trees or posts. It would be best to have the ground particularly prepared for this purpose, but turf is not durable enough, and a harder material has other disadvantages. This kind of running may be practised by single persons, or numbers, one following the other. A greater degree of swiftness, without neglecting the short turning, increases the difficulty considerably.

RUNNING IN A SPIRAL LINE.

He who leads, describes in running a spiral line; in the centre, he turns in the form of a hook, and returns through the interval between the lines of his followers; these have nothing to do, but to follow each one the man before him, and so on.

Another kind of running. The right foot is moved forward on the right side, the left brought up behind the right, then the right again; afterwards the left forward on the left side, the right brought up behind the left, and then the left again, and so on. In this way, always three steps are made on one side. This may be done by several who lay their hands upon each other's shoulders.

Running backwards, is of great use, but can be done only on level ground.

Running up a hill, the length and steepness of which gradually increases. A hill of considerable breadth is very convenient, so that a larger number can start at the same time.

Running, as well as walking, of every kind, may be practised with a load, increasing gradually in weight.

IV. LEAPING.

Leaping is to bound from the ground by means of a start, with one or both feet.

We shall mention those of the preparatory exercises which are of great importance for performing the different kinds of leaping.

 I. *Standing on tiptoe*, page 2.
 II. *Walking on tiptoe*, page 2.
 III. *Hopping*, page 2.
 IV. *Kicking*, page 2.
 V. *Crouching*, page 3.
 VI. *Hopping on one foot*, page 4.

OF LEAPS IN GENERAL.

Every leap has a *start* and *pitch*, both of which are to be executed by the toes alone, never by the whole foot.

In pitching, which always must be done with feet closed, the body should not form a straight line, but the shock is to be broken by bending the joints of the knees, hips, and feet, and by a slight inclination forwards.

Every leap may be performed

1. *from the spot* (standing jump),
2. *with a preparatory spring,*
3. *with running* (running jump).

The first and second kind are performed with feet closed.

1. In performing *the leap from the spot*, the person bends the knees quickly, then rises, drawing the knees towards the breast.

II. In performing *the leap with a preparatory spring*, the person stands one pace from the place of leaping, leaps, with his feet closed, upon that place, and then springs in the manner described in the preceding article.

These two kinds of leaping may be practised, at first, with the hands on the hips, to avoid an irregular position of the body, and unnecessary motions with the arms.

III. In performing *the leap with running*, this is to be observed. The leaper takes a run of twelve or fifteen paces. The run is not to be very swift, nor vehement; it serves only to increase the elasticity of the feet, and to accelerate the motion. The moment of reaching the place of leaping, one foot is placed upon it, the other thrown forwards; the first foot gives the start from the ground, and joins the other as quickly as possible, so that both feet are joined, before one half of the leap is accomplished. See pl. II, fig. 1.

It requires considerable practice, to measure the distance of the place of leaping, and to hit it exactly. Every one must become used to giving the start with either foot, and may run in a gallop in order to accomplish it.

Two particular kinds of leaping may be mentioned:

I. First kind. The feet are kept close, and the object is, to reach a certain point by the least number of leaps, without losing the balance.

II. Second kind or the leap-run. This run is distinguished from the common, by the perfectly perpendicular position of the body, or rather a slight inclination backwards, and by a very slight bending of the legs in stepping down;

for the rest, they are stretched out, so that the toes are turned to the ground. The body must rise after each step like a spring. No exercise increases the elasticity of the lower limbs more than this. Solid and level ground is required. Dexterity, swiftness, duration, and good appearance are principal objects.

Leaping is divided into two classes, according to the limbs which are used in accomplishing it, *Free* and *Mixed leaping*.

The free leap is performed by forcing the body through the air without the assistance of any other means, than that of the lower members. In mixed leaping, the hands and arms too are employed; it is divided into two branches, *Leaping with a pole*, and *Vaulting*, the latter of which, on account of its extensiveness and importance, will be treated of in a particular chapter.

A. FREE LEAPING.

The *free leap* may be performed as
1. *long leap*,
2. *high leap*,
3. *deep leap*.

1. LONG LEAP.

Instrument: a ditch, the banks of which are narrow at one end, and increasing in distance towards the other. The breadth ought not to increase more, than four inches per foot. A ditch from 4—16 feet in width, requires 36 feet in length. The bank from which the spring is made, must be solid, the opposite, soft and level. See pl. VII, fig. 7.

VARIATIONS OF THIS LEAP.

a. *forwards*;
b. *side-ways*,
   right,
   left;
c. *oblique*; the run is made straight,
   right,
   left.

d. turning; the leaper turns wholly around his own axis, which is, at first, to be practised on the spot.

e. backwards.

All these leaps may be performed *on the spot, with a spring,* and *with a run,* except the last, which can only be done on the spot. If performed without running, the hands may be placed upon the hips.

The best measure of the length of the leap, is the size of the leaper. A leap of once and a half the length of the body, may be expected from any person; of twice and a half, is a good jump; and of three times the length of the body, is an extraordinary one.

A means to gain certainty in leaping, is to leap, not singly, but in large numbers. A ditch of 30 feet in length, is required for a line of 12 leapers. The leap may be performed, at first, without, and gradually with, keeping step. Another similar kind of leaping is, to form a line with the best leaper at the head, who, followed by the rest at convenient distances, overleaps the windings of a rivulet, of different width and unequal banks.

2. HIGH LEAP.

Instrument: the leaping-stand consists of two posts, with holes bored through, and two iron pegs over which a cord, distended by two sand-bags fixed to each end of the cord, is placed so, that it will fall, or give way at the slightest touch. It is well, to have the cord colored; red is the color most easily perceived. The posts are six feet high, and eight feet distant from each other. The holes begin one foot above the ground, and are distant two inches from one another. See pl. VII, fig. *A.* and 6, *b.* The ground for the run must be solid and level in this kind of leaping, as well as in all others. It is better, if it descend a little, and rise again a short space from the place of springing.

VARIATIONS OF THIS LEAP.

They are the same as in the long leap. The best measure here also, is the size of the person exercising. The different degrees of height, may be conveniently arranged according to the following scale:

  to the height of the ankles,
    "   middle of the calves,
    "   knees,
    "   middle of the thighs,
    "   hips,
    "   lower ribs,
    "   pit of the stomach,
    "   neck or shoulders,
    "   chin,
    "   mouth,
    "   nose,
    "   eyes,
    "   forehead,
    "   crown of the head.

Most persons learn, by some practice, to leap as high as the pit of the stomach; few as high as the crown of the head.

To promote accuracy in leaping, the following exercises may be practised:

I. A number of 12 or 18 form a line; the first leaps over the string, and whilst he is joining the last of the line, the second leaps, and so on, until the whole line is in motion. At first the distance of the single leapers is ten paces, which gradually may decrease to five.

II. Lines of three or four are formed, who leap over the string at a time, at first without, afterwards with, keeping step. After some practice, the lines may be increased to 12, even to 25 leapers each.

LONG AND HIGH LEAP.

This leap is composed of the two preceding kinds. It may be practised on a common leaping-stand; but it is better to have a *moveable* one which is placed in the leaping-ditch. Thus the distance of the place of springing from the cord, is more easily fixed. This distance is to be changed, in order to perform the high leap either in the *first*, *middle*, or *last part* of the long leap.

3. DEEP LEAP.

Instrument: a flight of steps ten feet in height, the first being three feet above the ground, and each following rising one foot above the preceding. Every step must be at least a foot square. The place of descent must consist of, or at least be thickly covered with, loose sand.

Every leap is performed from the spot, without a run; an accurate descent, therefore, is the principal object. It must be performed so, that the toes touch the ground first; the knees must be ready to bend, the moment the feet touch the ground, in order to save the body from a sudden shock; on the other hand, the knees must not begin to bend, before the feet touch the ground, else they bend too hastily, and are apt to strike against the chin.

As to the measure, it is not advisable to exceed the depth of twice the length of the body.

DEEP AND LONG LEAP.

This leap is a combination of the first and third kinds, but it must be practised with great precaution, with a very slow increase of height and length. The flight of steps, if the place for descending is sufficiently large, may be used. A rivulet, or ditch with unequal banks, is suitable.

B. LEAPING WITH A POLE.

Instruments:

1. *The leaping-stand* has the same shape as that used for the free leap; but the posts must be ten feet high, and ten feet distant from each other. The holes begin two feet above the ground, and are three inches distant from one another. A step is to be fixed on the outside of each post, about two feet above the ground, for changing the pegs conveniently. See pl. VII, fig. *A*.

2. *Leaping-poles.* They are young, dried, and peeled fir stems, from 7—11 feet long, and of a proportionate

thickness, so that each one is strong enough to bear the gymnick. The lower thicker end is pointed, to avoid slipping. The ground is as described above, except that, about 1 1-2 feet from the cord, it must be made loose, for placing the pole safely, without danger of slipping.

Holding of the pole. One hand takes hold of the pole on the upper end, the thumb turned outwards, or upwards; the other below, the thumb turned in an opposite direction from that of the upper hand. The leap is more easily executed thus, than if the thumb of the lower hand is turned upwards. See pl. II, fig. 2.

Chief-points are these: the foot which is on the side of the lower hand, must always give the start; the left foot, if the left hand be below. The foot is placed several feet behind the pole, in proportion to the height of the leap, but at the same time with the pole. The legs rise on the side opposite to the foot giving the start (on the right side, if the left foot gave the start), and are thrown forwards as high as possible; the lower arm is stretched, the breast approaches near to the pole, and the body is turned, so that, in descending, it is looking towards the place of starting.

In order to learn the swinging of the feet, and preserving the equilibrium, the beginner must put his pole in a ditch, and leap from the spot; then take a short run, in order to learn the correct placing of the foot. The pole must be placed exactly in the direction of the leap, and then move in a perpendicular plane. Springing with the right and left foot, is soon to be learned; if the exact placing of the foot be somewhat difficult, the run in a gallop may be used. It is of importance to hold, during running, the pole in the direction of the leap, and horizontal; holding it obliquely and low, and suddenly turning it, at the moment of putting it down, interrupts the swing, and disturbs the equilibrium.

VARIATIONS OF THE LEAP.

I. *Long leap,* over the ditch,
    a. from the spot, for beginners,

18 FIRST SECTION.

b. with a run. A strong throwing forwards and stretching of the whole body, is altogether necessary for reaching some distance.

II. *High leap,* over the cord. This is the most difficult kind :

a. leaving the pole behind ; this is the common way.

b. taking it over ; this requires much practice.

The height of the fingers, when the arm is stretched, is the measure of a good leap. The complete turning of the leaper around his axis, is difficult in the high leap.

The long and high leap must be exercised on the ditch. The height may be estimated by the cord, placed as described above, page 15, but the latter will always be thrown down by the pole, since this cannot be left behind, as in the mere high leap.

III. *Deep leap,* only from the spot. The hands take hold of the pole as low as possible, and may slide still lower during the leap, in order to obtain a soft descent. The turning of the body is unnecessary in this leap.

The deep and long leap is very violent, and is, on this account, never to be made from a great height. The turning of the body is necessary in this leap.

An easy and convenient mode of leaping, with poles, is that *with two poles,* between which the gymnick leaps. It is, in its simplest form, too easy, and deserves to be practised only in the following manner, when it is very good for the joints of the back. Both poles are put in the middle of a ditch, three or four feet deep ; the pupil takes hold of them at the height of his shoulders, or the crown of his head, swings through them, bends the knees a little in touching the opposite bank, and pushes himself immediately back. This motion, continued, affords much exercise, especially if the ditch be from eight to ten feet wide.

All leaps may be performed, like the walks and runs, with and without a load ; but the arms and hands must not be incumbered.

V. VAULTING.

Vaulting, as we have seen above, belongs to the mixed leaps; the swing which the body receives by the spring of the feet, being assisted by the hands. The object, upon which the hands are placed, must be immoveable. But not only all leaps which carry the pupil, with the assistance of his hands, *upon* the machine, destined for this exercise, or *over* it, are considered as belonging to vaulting, but likewise all changes of position which he makes *on* it.

Vaulting, one of the most important exercises, has a salutary effect upon almost all parts of the body; it strengthens particularly the arms, legs, muscles of the belly and back, increases the agility, and improves the carriage.

Since *vaulting* is of so great importance, and, as an art, raised to so high a degree of perfection, it deserves particular lessons, like fencing. It is a very good exercise in winter, when, on account of the weather, the rest of the exercises must be suspended, and may be practised well enough in a large room, until there are houses appropriated for all the exercises.

Instrument: Vaulting-bar, or *vaulting-horse.*

Vaulting-bar is a machine, somewhat similar to a horse. It is for pupils of 15 years and more, 6 feet long, and 18 inches thick, towards the head decreasing a little, but on both ends perfectly round. It is good to have the horizontal diameter a little shorter, than the perpendicular. The croup is two feet, the saddle, with the holding pieces, one foot eight inches, and the neck two feet four inches. The holding pieces are 3 1-2 or 4 inches high, and 2 1-2 or 3 thick, the upper part must be round, the lower decreasing a little in thickness; they must not stand forth on the sides, by any means, but be thinned till they terminate in the surface of the bar; they should be made of good wood, inserted in the vaulting-bar, and made secure with long nails. The legs are fixed one foot from the hind end, and 20 inches from the forepart. Hind and fore legs deviate from the perpendicular direction, the latter forwards, and the former backwards, and towards the sides only so much, as not to project beyond the sides of the trunk more than four inches; or even less, if the legs are 6—8 feet in the ground. See pl. VII, fig. D.

Vaulting-horse. The croup rises towards the tail about one inch; the neck towards the head as much as the height of the saddle-holds (from 2—4 inches). The thickness increases in the croup to 20, and decreases in the neck to 12 inches. See pl. VII, fig. E.

The stuffing is done in the following manner. The whole trunk is covered with linen, upon which horse-hair is sewed; this is again covered with linen, and the whole with a well tanned horse-skin, without hair. The whole stuffing, made in this way, is 1-2 or 3-4 of an inch thick. Then the wooden saddle-holds, one inch and 1-4 thick, and three inches high, (see pl. VII, fig. F.) are fixed upon the trunk by means of three screws, eight or nine inches long, and 3-8 of an inch thick. A linen cushion, 1-2 or 3-4 of an inch thick, is placed upon the holds; the sides of the holds are filled with hair, and the whole covered with linen, and lastly with leather, like the whole horse. The leather, used for covering the holds, must be soft and strong.

Since the vaulting-horse must be made to be raised and lowered, the legs consist of pipes and slides, (see pl. VII, fig. G.). Each pipe is composed of four boards, 1 1-4 inches thick; the edges must be carefully removed, so that the whole receives a round shape. The pipes enter the trunk six or eight inches, and are driven in firmly; the lower end is held together by an iron ring. The slides are two inches square, and must exactly fit the pipes; therefore solid, and perfectly dry wood, is to be used. Holes, two inches distant from one another, and half an inch in diameter, are bored into them, beginning two inches above the ground. The pegs, put in the holes towards the inside, have a head, to prevent their sliding through. If not too expensive, it is better to have the slides of forged iron; such need to be only 1 1-2 or 1 3-4 inches square.

It is not adviseable to give the perfect shape of a horse to the vaulting-horse, on account of many sharp edges, which on a living horse are softened by flesh, and rendered harmless by their yielding to a shock.

The *vaulting-horse* must have the measures, above mentioned, after being covered. All corners, edges, nails standing forth, buckles, and seams, are to be avoided with the utmost care.

The saddle-cushion, which is placed upon every *vaulting-horse*, or *vaulting-bar with holds*, is half an inch thick, and reaches almost under the belly, where it is buckled.

If the *vaulting-horse* is made so, that it can be lowered to the distance of three feet eight inches from the ground, boys of ten years, as well as grown persons, may exercise on it.

The proper height of the horse for each one, is a little below his shoulders.

PREPARATORY EXERCISES.

We must here refer, once more, to the preparatory exercises, illustrated in the first chapter, most of them being of great importance for vaulting. We shall mention, severally, *those which may be practised on the horse, or without it;* besides *those which can be practised only on the horse.*

For performing the first five preparatory exercises, the pupil stands in an erect position, and with the feet closed, as near as possible to the vaulting-bar, without touching it; the hands take hold of the middle of the saddle-holds, the elbows turned upwards. See pl. I, fig. 12.

I. *Hopping*. Out of this position, the body is forced upwards, by means of a spring (preparatory exercise III, *b*. page 2,) and with the assistance of the hands so high, that the arms are stretched. See pl. I, fig. 13.

When the body has reached that height, it sinks, immediately, in a perpendicular line, touches the ground only for a moment, and then repeats the motion.

Common faults in this exercise are : falling forwards of the upper part of the body, throwing back the legs, not stretching the arms, pulling on the saddle-holds, and sinking of the elbows, instead of merely pressing downwards.

II. *Crouching.* By crouching, as a preparatory exercise for vaulting, we mean the preparatory exercise V, *b*, page 3. It is only in this exercise, performed on the vaulting-bar, that it is not possible to keep the upper part of the body perfectly perpendicular. The pupil, however, must avoid pushing the knees against the vaulting-bar, and must raise them over the saddle. See pl. III, fig. 1.

III. *Straddling.* See preparatory exercise VII, page 5. The gymnick should avoid, as much as possible, the falling forwards of the upper part of the body, and observe the stretching of the arms. See pl. III, fig. 2.

IV. *Raising one leg*, which can be practised here only sideways; preparatory exercise VIII, *b*. See pl. I, fig. 8. Care must be taken to keep the hanging leg in a perfectly perpendicular position, and prevent it from following the movement of the raised leg. The legs are raised alternately.

V. *Crossing;* preparatory exercise IX. See pl. I, fig. 10.

VI. *Pushing off.* The pupil hops up, lets the legs fall against the bar, as soon as the arms are stretched, and remains in rest. From this position, the legs are pushed off, both at a time, about a span from the bar, merely by a sudden shock, proceeding from the back, not by bending the knees. The same movement should be several times repeated. See pl. III, fig. 3.

VII. *Raising.* The pupil hops so high as to be in rest, and throws one leg over, so as to sit. He places both his hands upon the first saddle-hold, the thumbs forward, the fingers backwards, so that the elbows are as near to each other as possible, without being bent. Then he lets go the saddle with his legs, separating them widely, and keeping them straight, and is thus in a suspended position. From this position, he raises his body by drawing in the belly, as high as possible; then lowers himself again, by bending the elbows, so much, that he almost touches the saddle with his thighs. This movement should be repeated slowly, without any sudden start or spring. See pl. III, fig. 4.

VIII. *Swinging.* The pupil is in the suspended position, described in the preceding paragraph, the hands placed so near together, that they almost touch; he brings his legs into a swinging motion, drawing in the back, when swinging backwards, the belly, when forward. The higher and more uniform the swinging, the better it is. A gymnick, well practised, strikes his feet together, behind and before, the legs constantly kept straight. See pl. III, fig. 5.

IX. *Swinging with raising the knees.* The pupil who is in rest on the second saddle-hold, draws up his legs with one start, and puts them before him into the saddle; sinks them again, and puts them behind his hands, upon the croup. The soles must be firmly put down, especially forwards, and the feet closed. He who is able to perform this exercise from the saddle-hold, may practise it, putting his hands closely behind the second saddle-hold. See pl. III, fig. 6.

X. *Moving along, resting upon the hands,* in an upright position. The pupil places himself behind the vaulting-bar, puts his hands upon the croup, the lower part of the thumbs close together, the fingers of each hand turned to the outside, and springs so as to rest upon his hands, and so he moves on, with short grasps, along the whole vaulting-bar. The greatest difficulty is in passing the saddle-holds. See pl. IV, fig. 7.

RULES TO BE OBSERVED IN VAULTING.

1. In vaulting, as in all other gymnastick exercises, every thing must be practised right and left. A leap or vault is called a right one, if the right leg makes the most difficult,

first, or chief motion, or if the same, or the whole right side of the vaulter goes ahead. The side of the vaulting-bar does not decide.

2. A perpendicular position of the head and body, is to be sought, and observed, in all movements; likewise the stretching the joints of the knees and feet, if their bending is not requisite for the spring.

3. As in all leaping, the spring is made with, and the descent upon, the toes and balls of the feet.

4. If a vault is repeated, the vaulter, at every descent, is not allowed to remain on the ground, still less to spring several times, but must immediately force his body up again.

5. After mounting, the vaulter should rest on his thighs, not sit; thus only the body gains a solid, good position, and, in alighting, a firm support. This position is accomplished in this way: the upper part of the body is upright, the back drawn in, the joints of the hips, which, in sitting, are turned forwards, are stretched, so that the thighs hang down in a perpendicular line. Thus there is an empty space left between the body and saddle, large enough to admit the hand. If larger, the position is too forced. See pl. III, fig. 8.

6. Almost all vaults can be performed
    a. from the stand,
    b. with a spring,
    c. with a run.

a. In the first kind, the hands are placed upon the vaulting-bar, before the start, and, immediately after it, raise the body.

b. The spring is made, (except in a few vaults, performed with one hand) with legs and feet closed, but not too near the vaulting-bar.

c. The run should be no longer, than eight or ten paces, and terminates in the spring. Important, as well as difficult for the beginner, is the placing of the hands at the proper moment after the spring, especially in vaults from behind.

The spring should be made lightly and lowly; all the strength is to be laid out in the start.

The swing of the body, in consequence of the run, is shaken by the spring; the body, therefore, moves on, whilst the legs remain behind. This motion is increased by the start, which brings the shoulders of the vaulter at least over the croup. At this moment, after the start, both hands are, close together, far forwards, lightly, yet firmly put, but not struck, upon the bar; they assist the swinging of the body forwards; they give a strong push, the moment the shoulders have reached the place, where the hands were put. An accurate observance of this rule, renders it possible to leap over a vaulting-bar, seven or eight feet long.

All vaults are divided
    A. into simple,
    B. compound.

A. SIMPLE VAULTS.

They consist in the preparatory exercises, and simple movements, none of which is contained in the other. They are performed either
    a. from the side, or
    b. from behind.

a. VAULTS FROM THE SIDE.

I. *First mounting.* The pupil takes hold of the two saddle-holds, springs so as to rest on his hands, raises the right leg, till it forms a right angle with the left; leaves the grasp of his right hand, turns at the same time his right leg, and body, till the face is looking towards the horse's head; the right hand is put into the saddle, and the right leg closes gently.

First alighting. The right hand remains in the saddle; the right leg, and the body return at the same time, and the right hand reaches the second saddle-hold,* before the right

---

*We call the saddle-hold towards the head the first, that towards the croup, the second.

leg closes with the left. The body remains in rest for a moment, and then descends.

II. *Second mounting.* The pupil rests, as in the preceding exercise; the right hand suffers the right leg raised to pass through, and immediately takes hold again, so that the right leg gently touches the saddle.

Second alighting. The right hand is on the second saddle-hold; body and right leg return; the right hand is lifted up to let the right leg pass, and then renews its hold. The whole weight of the body is placed upon the left arm, during the movement.

It is best to mount on the right side, and alight on the left; then to mount on the left, and alight on the right.

Since it is difficult to turn the leg and body at the same time, a useful exercise is, when the hand has been placed in the saddle, not to suffer the leg to touch the saddle, but, after it has swung as far as the horse's neck, to return immediately to the other side.

The swing assists very much in taking back foot, body, and hand, at the same time. This exercise must be often repeated.

III. *Third vault.* The vaulter hops up so as to rest (see pl. I, fig. 13), and pushes back his legs (see pl. III, fig. 3); at this moment, the face is turned towards the head of the horse; the right leg is raised, and passes over the neck, so as to close, the left hand being lifted a little. During the movement the upper part of the body is straight; the weight of the body rests on the right arm; the left leg hangs straight down.

Alighting. The leg returns in the same way. The body, at first, is turned away a little from the horse, and, after the leg has passed over the first saddle-hold, again towards it. The pupil may alight by means of the right hand alone, which is, however, much more difficult.

This vault, like the two preceding, should be made twice in succession.

IV. *Fourth vault.* The beginning of the fourth vault is like that of the preceding, but, instead of one leg, both are raised forward. The body is turned forward, in a sitting position. After the left hand has suffered the legs to pass through, the right hand pushes off, and the vaulter descends, so as to stand at the first saddle-hold, on the right side of the horse, the face turned forward, the left hand on the first saddle-hold.

V. *Fifth vault.* The pupil, resting on his hands (see pl. I, fig. 13), pushes off his legs backwards, towards the croup of the horse, raising them closed up; the upper part of the body sinks towards the horse; the whole body, stretched out, passes over the horse. The right hand leaves the second saddle-hold; the left hand goes from the first saddle-hold to the second saddle-hold, and the descent is made on the side of the latter.

These five vaults described, are commonly exercised right, on the left side of the horse, and left, on the right side of the horse, so that at the termination of the vault, the pupil is turned forwards. But they must also be practised on the croup, and neck, and right, and left, on either side of the horse.

VI. *Sixth vault.* The vaulter mounts, and, resting with his hands on the first saddle-hold (in the manner described in the preparatory exercises, VII and VIII, page 22 and 23. See pl. III, fig. 5), swings several times, as described in the preparatory exercise VIII, page 23. The feet, when near together, are crossed, the body turns, and the hands push off, so that the body comes, at closing, into a situation opposite the first.

The crossing must be practised right and left. It is called right, when the shoulders are turned to the right, and, of course, the left leg passes under the right; left, when the shoulders turn to the left, and the right leg passes under the left. This exercise, too, is commonly made four times.

VII. *Seventh vault.* The hands are placed upon both saddle-holds (see pl. I, fig. 12), but the mounting is made upon the croup, closing with the calves, not with the thighs. The right leg alights, joins the left, and both swing closed, as far as over the neck; there they fall asunder, so as to close with the calves. The hands are changed, and the same movement made. Then, the left leg begins, and the same movement is made towards the right, so that, in the whole, the legs alight and close four times.

VIII. *Eighth vault.* The body rests, with the arms on both saddle holds (see pl. I, fig. 13), pushes back the legs (see pl. III, fig. 3), and crouches, so that the legs can pass through between the arms, and then be drawn back, in the same way, into rest. This is done twice, to and fro, the last time the hands push off, and the pupil descends, the legs perfectly straight. If this vault is performed with a run, it can be done only forwards. See pl. III, fig. 1.

IX. *Ninth vault.* After hopping, the right leg goes, in a turned position, around the right arm, and over the saddle; the left leg, and the body follow, so that, the left leg having passed over the croup, the vaulter closes, with his face towards the croup. Then he alights left (with the left leg over the neck).

X. *Tenth vault.* Resting on the arms. See pl. I, fig. 13. One leg is raised so as to pass over the saddle, between the arms; whilst the other is doing the same, the first returns, and so on, so that the feet always meet in the centre of the saddle.

XI. *Eleventh vault.* The gymnick rests on his arms (see pl. I, fig. 13), pushes off his legs (see pl. III, fig. 3), and raises them on each side (see pl. III, fig. 4). When the feet have reached the necessary height, that is to say, the top of the horse, the hands push off, and force the body over, so that the vaulter descends on the right side of the horse, with his back towards the horse. If performed with a run, legs and feet are not to touch the horse.

The *vaults from the side*, are commonly performed over the saddle, and from either side of the horse, right and left, so that the face is turned towards the head of the horse. But it is very exercising to perform them from any side, right and left, over the croup and neck, and frequently without taking hold of the saddle-holds.

The *vaults from the side*, are to be practised, at first, *resting on the hands*; then *from the ground*, those upon the horse, with a spring, those over it, with a run and spring.

There are four essential changes in the former kind:

a. The gymnick always rests on his hands, after hopping up, and before hopping down, after alighting, and before mounting.

b. The gymnick performs the mounting without stopping, but always rests on his hands, after alighting, or before hopping down.

c. The gymnick performs the alighting without stopping, but always rests on his hands, before mounting, and after hopping up.

d. The gymnick performs mounting and alighting, without stopping at all.

b. VAULTS FROM BEHIND.

I. *First vault.* Every vault, by which the vaulter comes into a suspended position, that is to say, where he rests solely on his arms, is comprised in this vault. The position of the hands is the same as in performing the *sixth vault from the side*, the fingers separated from the thumbs, and turned towards the body. See pl. III, fig. 5. It is practised first on the second saddle-hold, then on the first. Placing the hands, after the spring, far forwards, and then quickly taking hold of the saddle-hold, is altogether necessary.

It is connected with swinging off, and, by this, distinguished from the *eleventh vault from behind*. The legs are closed in swinging over the horse (see pl. III. fig. 5), and the whole body comes into a horizontal position. At this moment, the hands give a strong push, and turn towards the horse, yet close, and without touching, in order to prevent an accidental falling, or striking of the breast against the horse. A long and good swinging off is possible, besides the strong push of the hands, only by stretching perfectly the whole body, and especially the legs.

II. *Second vault.* The start is the same as in the preceding exercise. After the placing of the hands upon the croup, and during the rising of the body, the right leg passes forwards in an arch over the second saddle-hold (which motion is mentioned page 5, near the bottom, under preparatory exercise VIII); at the same time the right hand goes from the croup, over the right leg, passing to the second saddle-hold; when the right leg is between the arms, the left hand gives a push, and the gymnick descends on the left side of the horse, near to the second saddle-hold, with feet close; the right hand remains on the second saddle-hold. The legs are not allowed to touch the horse, during the whole vault. Left, the same movements with the opposite leg and hands; the descent is on the right side of the horse. After some practice, the gymnick may endeavor to descend near the first saddle-hold. The greater difficulty arises from the body being, for a longer time, without support; the swing, therefore, must be strong, but certain.

III. *Third vault.* Straight spring, not deviating towards the side on which the vault is to be made. Both legs close are forced up on the left side of the horse, and then the same movement as is described in *the third vault from the side* (page 26); that is to say, the right leg is raised, and passes over the horse, the left hand being lifted, so as to close. It is practised, at first, upon the croup, then into the saddle, at length upon the neck. The whole vault is performed without any interruption. The alighting, as described above, the right hand being placed upon the croup, the second, or first saddle-hold, according to the vault being made upon the croup, into the saddle, or upon the neck.

The body must be considerably inclined forwards, during the vault. The same is to be practised left.

IV. *Fourth vault.* Straight spring, not deviating to the right, the side on which the vault is to be performed. The legs are forced up on the right side of the horse. During the swing (or immediately at the commencement of the vault, which is, however, more difficult), the right hand takes hold of the second saddle-hold, the right leg passes over the horse, and swings, the breast turned towards the croup; the gymnick, improving the same swing, returns to his place of starting, the breast turned forwards. This likewise is to be performed left.

V. *Fifth vault.* The legs are forced up as in performing the preceding exercise, but on the left side of the horse, so that the left leg is in the saddle, the right leg on the croup (the second saddle-hold between the legs), the left hand on the second saddle-hold, the right hand upon the croup. The right hand gives a push, the body turns about the left arm; the right leg is raised backwards (see preparatory exercise VIII, page 5, near the bottom), passes over the neck, and the gymnick closes in the saddle, breast turned forwards. See pl. III, fig. 8. The right hand takes directly hold of the first saddle-hold, the thumb turned forwards, the left hand is placed upon the neck, and the pupil alights on the left side. This exercise is to be performed as swiftly as possible, yet accurately; it is likewise to be practised left.

VI. *Sixth vault,* or any leap, by means of which the vaulter comes, from behind, to stand upon the horse. The commencement is like that of the *first vault from behind,* the hands, after the spring, being placed upon the croup, and the body rising; but then the legs are quickly drawn up forwards, and placed upon the horse, before the hands, either upon the croup, the second saddle-hold, the saddle, the first saddle-hold, or neck. To rise quickly from this position, and firmly stand, is the chief thing. He who has great power of swinging, must come upon the horse with legs stretched, in proportion to the strength of his swing, in order to avoid falling forwards.

The *alighting* may be done:

a. by hopping off, from the croup, second saddle-hold, saddle, and first saddle-hold, not from the neck. The vaulter stands on the balls of his feet, springs, opens his legs, lest the feet meet some obstacle, and thus leaps backwards over the horse, closes his legs, and descends on the place of starting. The hands are stretched forwards. Before the gymnick hops off from the horse, he may hop to and fro, on the saddle-holds, but always on the ball of his feet.

b. or by the following vault:

The pupil, standing in the saddle, springs, turns, opens his legs so as to come gently to close, the face turned backwards. Then he makes the *sixth vault from the side* (page 27), and swings off from the first saddle-hold.

c. or by the following vault.

VII. *Seventh vault.* The gymnick, standing upon one saddle-hold on the balls of his feet, crouches, one hand between his feet on one, the other, on the other saddle-hold. In this position he hops from one saddle-hold to the other, always changing the hands, first to the right, then to the left side. Then he swings off, stretching and raising up the legs closed, the upper part of the body sinking towards the horse, and the whole body, stretched out, passing over the horse, (see *fifth vault from the side*, page 27), to the right, if the right hand is placed foremost, the left hand taking, during the descent, the place of the right; or to the left, if the left hand is placed foremost, the right hand taking, during the descent, the place of the left.

d. or by the following vault:

VIII. *Eighth vault.* The gymnick places his hands upon the horse's head, and swings over it, separating his legs.

IX. *Ninth vault.* Straight spring, not deviating towards the side on which the vault is to be performed. (See *third vault from the side*, page 26). The legs closed are forced up on the left side of the horse, pass over the horse to the right side; the descent is made near to the second or first saddle-hold, the left hand taking hold of the second or first saddle-hold, according to the length of the vault. The same is to be performed left.

X. *Tenth vault.* Straight spring, not deviating towards the side on which the vault is to be performed. The legs are forced up on the right side of the horse; during this swing, or, better, immediately at the commencement of the vault, the right hand takes hold of the second saddle-hold, the legs pass over the horse, and the gymnick descends on the left side, whilst the left hand takes the place of the right, the face turned backwards. The descent is made near the second or first saddle-hold.

In order not to interrupt the swing, it may, at first, be allowed to have the hands on the croup. A good performance of this vault, however, requires the placing the right hand upon the second saddle-hold, either at the commencement of the vault, which is best, or, at least, during the legs being forced up.

XI. *Eleventh vault*, or any leap from behind over the horse. But, since much practice is requisite for performing them, the *long leap* precedes. Every *long leap* brings the gymnick upon the horse, into the position of resting on his arms, and is, therefore, like the *first vault from behind* (page 29), at least in some respects; that is to say, the legs separate as much as possible, the hands leave the place where they were first placed, and stretch, as far as the body is carried by the swing, so that the body comes to rest upon the hands. If the swing is strong, they must bear at least as much as is necessary for the vaulter to close gently. Sitting down, or closing without placing the hands before, is not to be allowed at all.

There are two kinds of the *eleventh vault:*

a. forwards; the hands are placed in the saddle, if the horse be not too high. It is allowed to place them once more, upon the head, but it is better to do it only once. The descent is as in leaping (page 11), with a slight inclination forward.

b. backwards. During the spring, the vaulter turns face and breast backwards, draws in the belly, and holds his hands forwards.

If the *eleventh vault* has not carried the gymnick over, but only upon, the horse, the alighting is performed:

a. after the *long leap forwards,*

from the croup or saddle, in the common way, one hand being placed far, the other close before the body;

from the neck, the vaulter puts both his hands upon the horse's head, and swings over it, separating his legs (see the *eighth vault from behind,* page 32), the legs being kept straight.

b. after *the long leap backwards,*

from the croup, as in the preceding leap;

from the saddle likewise, or by the *third vault from the side* (page 26); that is to say, the gymnick places his hands upon both saddle-holds; the body, at first, is turned away a little from the horse, the leg, opposite to the hand which is before the body, passes over the horse, that hand being raised for a moment, then the body turns again towards the horse. Or alighting is performed by means of the hand, which is placed behind the body, alone;

from the neck by *swinging off;* the hands being placed upon the first saddle-hold, the fingers separated from the thumbs towards the body, the body, resting on the arms, swings off (see the *first vault from behind,* page 29 and 30).

Some more simple vaults follow, which are to be practised, though they are only variations of those enumerated.

I. *Mounting*, both hands on the first saddle-hold, and *alighting* in the same manner. The same vault is to be performed left. Compare the *first* and *second vaults from the side* (page 25, I, and 26, II).

II. The gymnick rests on his hands, upon both saddle-holds, with his back towards the horse; the right leg raised forwards, passes over the neck, the right hand being lifted, and closes gently. The same vault is to be performed left. Compare the *third vault from the side* (page 26, III).

III. The gymnick rests on his hands, upon both saddle-holds, with his back towards the horse; both legs raised forwards, pass over the neck, the right hand being lifted; descent on the other side. The same vault is to be performed left. Compare the *fourth vault from the side* (page 27, IV).

IV. The gymnick is resting on his hands, upon both saddle-holds; the right leg drawn up towards the breast (see preparatory exercise V c, page 4), passes over the saddle, and raised returns either over the croup, the right hand being lifted, or over the neck, the left hand being lifted. The same vault is to be performed left. Compare the *eighth vault from the side* (page 28, VIII, see pl. III, fig. 1).

V. The gymnick, taking hold of both saddle-holds, and drawing up his knees towards the breast (see pl. III, fig. 1), comes to stand upon the saddle. Compare the *eighth vault from the side* (page 28, VIII).

Another kind is from behind. After run and spring, the hands are placed upon the croup, the knees drawn up, and placed between the hands, so that the gymnick comes to stand upon the croup.

VI. Compare the *sixth vault from the side* (page 27, VIII), with the three following vaults.

a. The gymnick, in a riding position, is resting on his hands; the legs swing forwards, and cross when they have reached the top of the horse, the left hand being lifted; or the legs swing backwards, and cross, the right hand being lifted which is, however, much more difficult.

b. The gymnick is sitting in the saddle, both hands are placed on the second saddle-hold, the legs are raised forwards, and crossed.

c. The gymnick is sitting in the saddle, both hands are placed on the first saddle-hold, the belly leans against the first saddle-hold, the legs are raised backwards, and crossed.

It is evident that these three vaults, by crossing the legs, effect a reversing of the position, but in a different manner from one another.

VII. Compare the *sixth vault from behind* (page 31, VI), with these vaults.

After the run and spring from behind, the hands are placed upon the croup, whilst the body is rising, the legs are quickly drawn up forwards, and are placed upon the horse before the hands, upon the saddle; from this position

a. the left hand is placed upon the first saddle-hold, the right upon the neck, the legs swing from the saddle over the neck, whilst the body, the back turned upwards, is stretching itself, like the *fifth vault from the side* (page 27, V). The same vault is to be performed left.

b. The right hand is placed upon the first saddle-hold, the left upon the neck, the legs swing from the saddle forwards, over the neck, the body being in a sitting position, like the *fourth vault from the side* (page 27, IV). The same vault is to be performed left.

c. The vault described under paragraph VII, or the *sixth vault from behind*, performed on *one* foot.

VIII. Both hands on the first saddle-hold, the fingers forwards, the thumbs towards the belly, the legs, closed on one side, are thrown over to the other side; this movement is repeated several times.

It is much easier, to place the hands behind, upon the second saddle-hold.

Many of the vaults mentioned, both from the side, and from behind, may be performed with one hand, and so we get the class of

FENCING-VAULTS, or VAULTS WITH ONE HAND.

They have the peculiarity, that most of them, except the *sixth, eighth,* and *eleventh vaults from behind* (page 31, 32 and 33), are performed with *one foot,* as well as one hand. Position and run, is taken obliquely, for performing the vaults from the side.

I. *Mounting:*
    with the left hand, and right foot,
    with the right hand, and left foot.

II. *The third vault from the side* (page 26), *and the third vault from behind* (page 30):
    with the left hand, and right foot,
    with the right hand, and left foot.

In both vaults (I and II), that foot which does not execute the vault, makes the spring.

III. The *fourth vault from the side* (page 27), and the *ninth vault from behind* (page 32 and 33):
    right, the left foot making the spring,
    left, the right foot making the spring.

IV. The *fifth vault from the side* (page 27), and the *tenth vault from behind* (page 33):
    right, with the left foot making the spring,
    left, with the right foot making the spring.

V. *Fifth vault,* between the *fourth* and *eighth vaults from the side* (page 27 and 28):
    right, whilst the left foot springs,
    left, whilst the right foot springs.

A pure *eighth vault from the side* (page 28), which is the same as a common high leap without a pole (see page 14, and pl. II, fig. 1), with a straight run and spring, may be performed, if the horse is pretty low.

VI. The *sixth vault from behind* (page 31 and 32):
    with the right hand,

with the left hand.
VII. The *eighth vault from behind* (page 32) :
   with the right hand,
   with the left hand.
VIII. The *eleventh vault from behind* (page 33) :
   forwards,
   backwards ;
   with the right hand,
   with the left hand.

In these three last vaults, the run and spring is straight, not oblique, as in the first.

B. COMPOUND VAULTS.

The *compound vaults* may be multiplied very much ; but the following are the most distinguished :

I. *First vault.* The gymnick performs the *second mounting (second vault from the side*, page 26, II), with the right leg ; that is to say, the right leg raised, passes over the horse, the right hand being lifted for a moment, and, without touching the horse, passes, a second time, over the horse, the left hand being lifted (alighting after the *third vault from the side*, page 26, III) ; descent; the right leg raised passes over the horse, the left hand being raised *(third vault from the side*, page 26, III), passes, a second time, over the horse, the right hand being lifted *(second alighting*, page 26, II), so that the right leg has described two semicircles. The same vault is to be performed with the left leg.

II. *Second vault.* The gymnick takes hold of both saddle-holds, and forces his legs upon the croup, as if to perform the *fourth vault from the side ;* then the right leg performs the *ninth vault from the side* (page 28, IX), that is to say, it is raised, and passes over the saddle, so that the gymnick comes to sit in the saddle ; the left leg performs the alighting by passing over the horse, the right hand being lifted (alighting after the *third vault from the side*, page 26, III). The same vault is to be performed with the left leg.

III. *Third vault.* The left hand is on the second saddle-hold, the right on the croup; the right leg is raised, and swings over the horse, during which movement the right hand goes from the croup upon the second saddle-hold, the thumb turned forwards; whilst the right leg is returning in the same way, the left hand passes over to the first saddle-hold; descent; then both legs are raised forwards, the body is turned forwards, in a sitting position; the left hand suffers the legs to pass through, and the gymnick descends on the other side (see the *fourth vault from the side*, page 27, IV). The same exercise is to be performed with the left leg.

Another kind. The gymnick passes with his right leg over the neck, the left hand being lifted (see the *third vault from the side*, page 26, III), but instead of closing, he returns immediately in the same way (alighting after the *third vault from the side*, page 26, III); descent; then the gymnick performs either the *fourth* or the *fifth vault from the side*, (page 27, IV, and V).

IV. *Fourth vault.* One hand on each saddle-hold; the right leg is raised, and swings over the horse, the right hand remaining on the second saddle-hold, and the left leg close on the saddle; the right leg returns in the same way, and then the gymnick performs the *fourth vault from the side*, right (page 27, IV), that is to say, the legs are raised on the left side, the body turns to the left in a sitting position; after the left hand has suffered the legs to pass through, the right hand pushes off, and the vaulter descends on the opposite side of the horse, the face turned towards the left, the left hand on the first saddle-hold.

Or the gymnick, instead of the *fourth vault from the side*, performs the *fifth vault from the side*, left (page 27, V); that is to say, he forces his legs up backwards, towards the neck of the horse, the upper part of the body sinks towards the horse, the whole body, stretched out, passes over the horse; the left hand leaves the first saddle-hold, the right hand goes from the second to the first saddle-hold, and the descent is made on the opposite side of the horse, near the first saddle-hold.

The same vault is to be performed left, and then the *fourth vault from the side*, left, or the *fifth vault from the side*, right.

V. *Fifth vault.* The left leg is raised towards the croup of the horse, and swings over the horse, the right hand being lifted, but does not close; the left leg is forced backwards over the horse's neck, the left hand being lifted; and then the preceding vault, right. The same vault is to be practised, beginning with the right leg.

VI. *Sixth vault.* One hand on each saddle-hold, the legs are forced up, forwards upon the neck (as if to perform the *fourth vault from the side*, right), the right hand passes to the first saddle-hold, near the left; the left leg is raised forwards towards the croup, and passes over the horse, so that the gymnick comes to sit in the saddle, face towards the neck; then *second alighting* (page 26, II), the left leg passing over the croup, the left hand being lifted; then the legs are forced up, forwards upon the croup, the right hand passes from the first to the second saddle-hold, the left leg is raised forwards towards the neck, and passes over the horse, so that the gymnick comes to sit in the saddle, face towards the croup; then *second alighting*, the left leg passing over the neck, the left hand being lifted. The whole terminates with the *fourth vault from the side* (page 27, IV), right, the legs being raised forwards, towards the horse's head, the body, in a sitting position, passing over the horse, the left hand being lifted, and descending at the first saddle-hold. The same vault is to be practised left.

VII. *Seventh vault.* Both hands are placed upon the second saddle-hold, the thumb of the right hand turned forwards, that of the left hand backwards; the right leg raised passes over the horse, but without closing; both legs straddling are raised; the body wheels, over the second saddle-hold, around the arms as axis, the hands following the movement. The same vault is to be practised left.

VIII. *Eighth vault.* Both hands are placed upon the second saddle-hold, the thumb of the right hand turned forwards, that of the left hand backwards; the right leg raised passes over the horse, swings back without closing; as soon as it has joined the left leg, both are raised forwards, and the body turned forwards, in a sitting position, passes over the horse. The latter part of the vault is the *fourth vault from the side,* (page 27, IV), the hands being placed upon one saddle-hold. The same vault is to be practised left.

IX. *Ninth vault.* Both legs are forced up, forwards, upon the croup, as if to perform the *fourth vault from the side,* left (page 27, IV); both legs return in the same way, are immediately raised forwards, and the body, in a sitting position, passes over the horse, the left hand being lifted *(fourth vault from the side,* right, page 27, IV).

X. *Tenth vault.* One hand on each saddle-hold, the right leg raised swings over the horse, and back, the left leg passes over the horse, the left hand being lifted *(second mounting,* page 26, II, without closing), passes again over the horse, the right hand being lifted (alighting after the *third vault from the side,* page 26, III); then the same movement performed by the right leg; after this the right leg is raised forwards, and passes over the horse, the left hand being raised *(third vault from the* side, right, page 26, III); alighting.

XI. *Eleventh vault.* Both legs are raised up, forwards, to the neck of the horse, the body is turned forwards, in a sitting position; the left hand suffers the legs to pass through towards the right (so far the vault is exactly the same with the *fourth vault from the side,* page 27, IV), the movement of the legs is continued, the right hand being lifted, and the descent is made on the same spot, whence the gymnick started. The whole movement, from the beginning to the end, is to be performed without the least interruption, the hands being promptly lifted. The same vault is to be performed left.

XII. *Twelfth vault*. The left hand is placed upon the second saddle-hold, the right hand upon the croup, the legs are raised over the croup, as if to perform the *fourth vault from the side*, left (page 27, IV), but then the movement of the legs is continued, the right hand yielding, the left hand following the movement of the body, without loosening the grasp, over the saddle, the gymnick turning his back upwards, whilst passing over the saddle, so that the descent is made, whence the start. The same vault is to be performed left.

There are two things constantly to be borne in mind in using the descriptions in this chapter on *Compound Vaults*.

Whenever it is not particularly expressed in which posture the gymnick is in the commencement of the vault, the posture described above, (page 21, see pl. I, fig. 12), is to be understood, that is to say, the gymnick stands on the left side of the horse, having the horse's head on his left, the croup on his right, and taking hold of the first saddle-hold with his left hand, of the second with his right.

Whenever a vault is mentioned as being to be performed left also, not only the first movement of the vault is meant to be performed with the opposite member (hand or leg), but the following likewise. The words: *the same exercise is to be performed left*, are, therefore, to be understood mutatis mutandis.

C. CONTINUED VAULTS.

The *Continued Vaults* consist in performing repeatedly the same vault, and require, therefore, strength and perseverance in a high degree. It is to be remembered, never to stop; if it should be difficult to start immediately after the descent, it is allowed to make a spring, and then start.

I. *Fourth vault from the side* (page 27, IV).

a. Both legs are raised forwards, up to the neck of the horse, the body is turned forwards, in a sitting position.

After the left hand has suffered the legs to pass through, the right hand pushes off, and the gymnick descends, so as to stand at the first saddle-hold, the face turned forwards, the left hand on the first saddle-hold;

b. the same vault left, over the neck of the horse;

c. the same vault left, over the croup of the horse; and lastly

d. the same vault right, over the croup of the horse.

Thus, *the fourth vault from the side*, is performed four times in succession, twice over the neck, right and left, and twice over the croup, left and right.

Another mode of continuing this vault is:

a. right over the neck of the horse;

b. right over the croup of the horse;

c. left over the croup of the horse;

d. left over the neck of the horse.

Thus, the *fourth vault from the side*, is performed four times in succession, twice right, over the neck and croup of the horse, and twice left, over the croup and neck of the horse.

A *third* mode of continuing this vault is:

a. right over the croup, left over the saddle, right over the neck;

and from the right side of the horse;

b. left over the croup, right over the saddle, left over the neck.

II. *Fifth vault from the side* (page 27, V).

a. The gymnick, resting on his hands, pushes off his legs backwards, towards the croup of the horse, raising them closed up; the upper part of the body sinks towards the horse, the whole body stretched out, passes over the horse; the right hand leaves the saddle-hold, the left goes from the first to the second saddle-hold, and the descent is made on the side of the latter;

b. the same vault, left, over the croup;

c. the same vault, left, over the neck;

d. the same vault, right, over the neck.

Thus, the *fifth vault from the side*, is performed four times in succession, twice over the croup, right and left, and twice over the neck, left and right.

Another mode of continuing this vault is:

a. right over the croup of the horse;
b. right over the neck of the horse;
c. left over the neck of the horse;
d. left over the croup of the horse.

Thus, the *fifth vault from the side*, is performed four times in succession, twice right, over the croup and neck of the horse, and twice left, over the neck and croup of the horse.

A *third* mode of continuing this vault is:

a. right over the croup, left over the saddle, right over the neck

and from the right side of the horse:

b. left over the croup, right over the saddle, left over the neck.

If the *fourth* and *fifth vaults from the side*, are compounded, a great number of variations may be made.

III. *Eighth vault from the side* (page 28, VIII; see pl. III, fig. 1.):

The gymnick draws up the knees towards the breast, so that the legs can pass through between the arms; the hands push off, and the descent is made on the right side of the horse.

a. from the left to the right, and from the right to the left side of the horse,

over the saddle,
over the croup,
over the neck.

b. from the left to the right side of the horse, over the croup; from the right to the left side of the horse, over the saddle; and from the left to the right side of the horse, over the neck; or the reverse.

IV. *Eleventh vault from the side* (page 28, XI, see pl. III, fig. 2.):

The gymnick raises his legs, separated, on each side; when the feet have reached the top of the horse, the hands push off, and force the body over, so that the vaulter descends on the right side of the horse, with his back towards the horse.

If this vault should be continued, it would require great exactness in performing, and two persons for assisting.

D. DOUBLE VAULTS.

The *Double Vaults*, and still more the *Threefold Vaults*, require particular accuracy in the gymnick, in order to perform them in unison with his fellow gymnicks.

I. *First and second mounting* (page 25, I, and 26, II): A mounts left upon the neck, B right upon the croup.

II. The *third vault from the side* (page 26, III): A performs it right upon the neck, B left upon the croup, so that both sit back to back.

III. The *fourth vault from the side* (page 27, IV): A performs it right over the neck, B left over the croup, so that in passing over the horse, and descending, they are turned with their backs against each other.

IV. The *fifth vault from the side* (page 27, V): A performs it left over the neck, B right over the croup, so that in passing over the horse, and descending, they are turned with their faces towards each other.

V. The *eighth vault from the side* (page 28, VIII): A performs it over the neck, B over the croup.

VI. A performs the *third vault from the side* (page 26, III) upon the saddle, B the *sixth vault from behind* (page 31, VI), upon the croup, places his hands on A's shoulders, and, thus, swings off backwards from the horse. A must take care to support the upper part of his body by resting his arms firmly upon the first saddle-hold, and to bend his head forwards.

VII. A performs the *third vault from the side* (page 26, III) upon the saddle; B the *first vault from behind*, (page 29, I) upon A's shoulders, and swings backwards off from them, over the croup of the horse.

VIII. The *sixth vault from behind* (page 31, VI): A performs it from before upon the neck, B from behind upon the croup; both hop, A upon the first, B upon the second saddle-hold; either both hop off from the horse (alighting after the *sixth vault from behind*, page 32, *d*), or A alone, and B performs the alighting after the *sixth vault from behind*, (page 32, *b*).

IX. The *first vault from behind* (page 29, I): A performs it from before upon the neck, B from behind upon the croup.

E. THREEFOLD VAULTS.

The *Threefold Vaults* are executed by three gymnicks, at a time.

I. The *eighth vault from the side* (page 28, VIII, see pl. III, fig. 1): A performs it over the neck, B over the saddle, C over the croup. B alone makes use of the saddleholds.

II. A performs the *third vault from the side* (page 26, III) right upon the neck, B the same left upon the croup, and C the *eighth vault from the side* over the saddle, (page 28, III, see pl. III, fig. 1.). C alone makes use of the saddle-holds.

III. A performs the *fourth vault from the side* (page 27, IV) right over the neck, B the same left over the croup, C the *eighth vault from the side*, over the saddle (page 28, VIII, see pl. III, fig. 1.). C alone makes use of the saddle-holds.

IV. A performs the *sixth vault from behind*, from before upon the neck, B from behind upon the saddle, C upon the croup. A and C alight by means of the *eighth vault from behind*, A from the neck, C from the croup; B performs the alighting after the *sixth vault from behind* (page 32, *b*).

This vault may be altered into one performed by four persons, if one performs before A, the *eleventh vault from behind*, over the horse.

F. FREE VAULTS.

The *Free Vaults* are performed only *over* the horse, not upon it, and without touching it at all. We are well aware that they, on this very account, properly belong to the *Free Leaps*, according to our own definition above (page 13); but since one of them cannot be performed on any other instrument, so as to show the whole movement, except on the horse, we insert them here.

I. *High leap* with both legs closed, from the side, over the saddle.

The following vault may serve as a preparatory exercise for the *high leap*. After the run and start, the right leg is thrown over the saddle, without making use of the hands, so that the gymnick comes to sit in the saddle, the face turned forwards. The same vault is to be practised left.

II. The *eleventh vault from behind* (page 25, XI), or *long leap*, from behind, over the horse, without the assistance of the hands; the start is made with one foot. Straddling is difficult in performing this leap.

The chapter on Vaulting, is, strictly taken, finished, but some more exercises, which commonly are performed on the horse, or vaulting-bar, may here be mentioned.

a. EXERCISES WITH THE HEAD FOREMOST.

I. The *eleventh vault from behind* (page 25, XI), upon the saddle, both hands placed upon the first saddle-hold, the belly leaning upon the saddle, the gymnick turns over to the right, or left side of the horse.

II. The gymnick performs the *eighth vault from the side* (page 28, VIII, see pl. III, fig. 1), yet does not descend, but remains resting on his arms; the back leans against the horse, the hands take firm hold, and the gymnick turns over backwards.

III. The gymnick sits upon the second saddle-hold, falls backwards, taking hold of the horse's tail, so as to stand behind the horse.

IV. The gymnick stands in the saddle, places one foot upon the neck, the hands upon the head, and thus wheels over.

V. Run from the side; the hands take hold of both saddle-holds, the gymnick turns over, and descends on the other side of the horse, with the back towards the horse.

b. EXERCISES IN A SUSPENDED POSITION.

I. The body, stretched out, rests horizontally upon the elbow of the right arm, the hand of which is placed upon the second saddle-hold; the left hand, placed upon the first saddle-hold, supports, or placed upon the second saddle-hold, which is more difficult, or does not support at all, which is the most difficult.

II. The gymnick moves around, in the position described in the preceding exercise, and swings off, or turns over.

LEAP-FROG.

The following leap, commonly called leap-frog, is included in *vaulting*.

Position of the person, standing:

one foot before the other, both turned outwards, the heel of the forward foot before the toes of the other;

the leg, which is behind, bent in the knee, the other straight, knee touching knee;

the hands rest upon the knees, the elbows stretched and close by the body;

the head pressed down upon the breast.

The leap may be executed by a large number. All stand at equal distance, one behind the other, in a straight, or curved line; the last begins to leap, after he has passed over two, the last but one begins. The distance of the single ones depends upon the skill of the leapers, whether they require a long, or short run, or none at all. It is to be practised only by persons of the same size, age, and strength.

Vaulting must always be practised under the superintendance, and direction of an experienced person, who is constantly ready to afford the necessary help. This help is right only, if it prevents falling, and increases the swing without interrupting the motion.

VI. BALANCING.

Balancing is preserving the equilibrium in rest, as well as in motion.

Instruments:

1. *Lying bar*, a mast of smooth wood, as long as possible, but not thicker than eight inches at the large end, lying on the ground.

2. *Suspended bar*, a slender straight pine tree, without knots; the longer it is, the better; it is not well to have it less than 40 feet long, and 10 inches thick, at the large end. It is supported at the large end, and at some distance from the small, between two pair of strong posts, upon iron pegs which can be fixed at different heights. Care must be taken that the vibrating motion of the mast be neither too great, nor too small. Much depends, in this respect, upon the distance at which the two pair of posts are fixed from each other. See pl. VII, fig. N.

3. *Small bar*, 16 feet long, and of a proportionate thickness, laid across an excavation, from one to two feet deep.

Some other instruments, but of less importance, are:

4. A *post*, reaching forth from the ground about one foot, and three inches in diameter.

5. A *plank*, erected on the edge, and secured at each end.

6. A *board* or *plank*, narrow, and with a smooth surface, across an excavation, from one to two feet deep.

The *ground*, around these instruments, must consist of, or be covered with, loose sand.

PREPARATORY EXERCISES.

I. *Standing on one leg*, the other is stretched out forwards, or backwards, bent, placed upon the hand or arm, raised up to the chin, one or both hands assisting, and the head bending downwards; it is well to throw, or catch something, to put on, or off the coat, all of which oblige the body to turn to different sides. The knee of the leg standing must not be bent.

II. *Walking on the juncture of two boards,* or on any other straight line, the feet turned outwards.

III. *Walking with legs stretched far, and raised high.* The slower the raising of the foot, and the stepping down, the more difficult it is for the beginner; arms and hands must hang down.

EXERCISES.

The following exercises are, at first, to be practised upon the *lying*, then upon the *suspended bar*.

I. *Balancing walk*, from the large to the small end; the feet outwards, step upon the sole, mouth shut, eyes directed upon the bar;

    a. forwards,

    b. backwards,

    c. over some obstacle, as a hat placed upon the bar, or a rod, or a string, held up.

Turning at the small end, is especially to be practised.

After some skill in this kind of walking has been acquired, walking, with the arms folded, is to be practised.

II. *Passing by one another.* Each person puts his right foot against the other's right, or the left against the left, takes hold of the other's arms, and steps by with the other foot turned inwards.

III. *Taking up something*, as a hat, from the small end.

IV. *Sitting down*, and *rising*, without the help of the hands.

V. The gymnick sits in a riding position, at the small end, rests the weight of his body on his arms, draws up both legs on the bar, either behind the hands (which is easier), or before the hands (which is the more difficult way), and stands upright; then stoops down, places his hands on the bar, and recovers the first position.

VI. *Raising one foot* towards the mouth, first on the large end, afterwards on those parts of the bar which are subject to a stronger vibration.

VII. *Balancing combat*, when two persons, standing opposite to each other, strive to remove each other from the bar by slight strokes.

Posture.

The feet, at a moderate distance from each other, are turned outwards, the right foot considerably bent, the left stretched. The arms are raised, as if to embrace something.

The strokes must be directed solely against hands, arms, and shoulders, and given with the palm of the hand. The hands are to be withdrawn, only when the adversary strikes. Leaning forwards, or backwards, with dexterity, avoiding the stroke of the adversary, and striking directly after, are chief advantages.

There are some other exercises which may be briefly mentioned here, because they are founded on the same principle as *balancing*, treated of above, viz. preserving the equilibrium. These exercises are *Walking on Stilts*, and *Scating*.

A. WALKING ON STILTS.

Instruments:

A pair of *stilts*. A stilt consists of a square pole, the sharp corners of which are rounded off, provided with a step; the step must be secured to the pole in such a manner as not to impair the firmness of the latter. The poles are of different height, from five to ten feet. The steps are from one to five feet from the ground. The upper part of the pole, from the step, is in proportion to the size of the person using the stilts; it should, however, reach nearly to the crown of the head, in order to avoid injuring the armpits.

Holding of the stilts. The stilts lean against the shoulders, either from before, the thumbs upwards, or from behind, the thumbs turned downwards. The former mode of holding allows a more upright posture of the body, but is more fatiguing to the hands and arms; the latter allows more freedom of motion, but frequently induces the gymnick to bend forwards.

The feet are placed upon the steps, with the balls, rather than with the hollow of the foot, like the placing the foot in the stirrup. Care must be taken, not to remove the step from the foot during walking.

I. *Walking;* a firm, and upright posture, is a principal object.

II. *Running :*

    a. trotting, which is only a quickened walking;

    b. galloping, always the same foot stepping first; it must be practised right, and left.

III. *Hopping on one stilt.* The gymnick takes one stilt from beneath the foot, and places it upon his shoulder, and hops with the other, bearing the whole weight.

    a. on the spot,

    b. moving from the place

        forwards,

        backwards,

        laterally, to the right and left.

IV. *Ascending* and *descending* steps; should be practised with the utmost caution, and never on a high flight of steps;

a. with both feet,
b. hopping on one stilt.

B. SCATING.

Instruments:

A pair of *scates.* It must be unnecessary to describe scates, as they are so well known to the people of those parts of the country who have occasion for their use. We shall, therefore, confine ourselves to a few remarks.

As to the *thickness* of the steel-piece, it is well to have it, at least, one-fifth of an inch thick; if it be thinner, it is not only apt to break, but also to cut deeper into the ice, than is necessary, or expedient.

The steel-piece of most scates, is *hollow.* Such scates are convenient on this account, because the edges, which are, of course, sharper, prevent sliding, in moving the foot towards the side. Beginners, at least, should make use of this kind of scates. Those who have acquired some familiarity with the exercise, may use scates with *flat* steel-pieces, which are preferred by many good scaters, and indeed accelerate the motion.

It is of importance that the steel-piece is not too low; it should be at least *three fourths of an inch high.* If it is lower, the scater is apt, when moving his foot to the side, to touch the ice with the wooden part of the scate, and thus to check his movement, if not occasion a fall.

As to the *size* of the scates, they should suit the length of the foot; they are very inconvenient, if so long, that the wooden part extends beyond the sole.

Mode of fastening.

There are various modes of *fastening* the scates to the feet. It might be difficult to decide in favor of any particular kind, provided that it answers these *three* purposes:

to keep the scate close to the foot, so as to prevent its clapping, at every step;

to keep the scate close to the foot, so as to prevent its moving to the right or left, either below the ball, or the heel of the foot;

to be fastened in such a manner, as not to prevent the free circulation of the blood through the foot, or even the free motion of the joint of the heel.

If there is, really, a difference between the modes of fastening scates, combining these three qualities, it is owing to the different shape of the foot, rather than to any thing else.

PREPARATORY EXERCISES.

I. *Standing on scates,* without losing the balance, in consequence of the joints of the feet turning over.

II. *Gliding,* the smooth motion on the scates over the ice;

    a. on both feet; the gymnick, standing on both feet, the scates parallel, is gently pushed along by another person, to accustom him to preserve the equilibrium, during the motion.

    b. on one foot, alternately; the whole weight is to be placed upon the foot which is to glide, the other foot pushing slightly from the ice, and so on, one foot after the other.

There are two precautions to be observed in this preparatory exercise: to *lean forwards,* in order to prevent falling backwards, and *not to turn the feet outwards,* in order to prevent the legs from separating in a straddling posture.

VARIATIONS OF SCATING.

There are two kinds of movements, in *straight,* and *circular* lines.

I. *Scating in straight lines.* This is the preparatory exercise II, *b,* brought to perfection. The right foot is foremost, almost straight forwards, the whole weight of the body resting on it, the knee bent; the left foot, behind the right, turned outwards, pushes off, the whole steel pressed against the ice, and forming right angles with the plane of the right foot; after the left foot has pushed off, it draws up near the right, as near the ice as possible; whilst the right foot continues its gliding motion, the right knee gradually stretches, and the upper part of the body erects itself. The longer the gliding on one foot, the better. When the motion becomes too slow, but not before, the left foot, hitherto quiet, close to the right, is brought forwards, and placed almost straight forwards, the right foot turning the toes outwards, and pushing off.

All motions of the body, and shaking of the arms and hands, are to be avoided. Crossing the arms before the breast, or on the back, is of use to render the body steady.

Stopping is effected, when the gymnick, gliding along on both feet, in a parallel position, leans slightly forwards, and raises the toes a little.

A means to accustom to long and uniform steps, is to form a line of several gymnicks, with their hands placed on one another's shoulders, and moving along, with keeping step.

II. *Scating in circular lines.* The movement of the foot forms, instead of straight, or nearly straight, lines, *quadrants* or even *semicircles*. The movement in circular lines, is performed

    a. outwards,
    b. inwards.

a. Scating in circular lines outwards. The movements of the feet are the same as in scating in straight lines, but the carriage of the body is different. While the left foot pushes off, the gymnick inclines his body stretched towards the right side, towards the centre of the quadrant, or semicircle which he is going to describe, bending the joint of the right hip, and raising, after the pushing off, the left foot over the right. Towards the close of the circular line, the body begins to incline to the left side, or towards the centre of the quadrant or semicircle, next to be described; the left foot is put down, and the right pushes off.

Scating in straight lines, with the body perfectly straight, and the foot, which pushed off, raised over the other gliding, may serve as a preparatory exercise for scating in circular lines. After having acquired some certainty in this motion, the gymnick may begin to incline, gradually, to the side, opposite to the foot pushing off.

This kind of *scating in a circular line*, may be performed *backwards*.

b. Scating in circular lines inwards. This is performed by a carriage of the body, in general the reverse of that described in the preceding exercise *a*. When the left foot has pushed off, the gymnick inclines towards the left, and brings up his left foot near the right. Towards the close of the line, the left foot is put down, the right pushing off, and the body inclining towards the right.

This exercise does not appear so dangerous as the preceding, because the leg pushing off is on the side to which the body inclines, and may serve as a support.

The length of the radius of the circular line, may be ten feet, and increase to fifteen or twenty, or decrease to five and less. The movement with the former radius is more graceful, that with the latter considered more difficult.

III. To the two principal kinds of scating, described under I and II, several others may be added, which, as to their principle, belong to either of the two.

a. Scating in a serpentine line. The gymnick, standing upright, the scates parallel, not raised from the ice, turns, alternately to the right and left, the right and left foot alternately giving an almost imperceptible pressure against the ice-plane, and thus producing the advancing motion.

b. Scating in a straight line towards the side. In the midst of a swift course, the gymnick turns suddenly the toes of both feet so far outwards, that the scates form one straight line, and glides along in this posture. Most are obliged to bend the knees in order to bring the feet into a straight line; though it cannot be entirely avoided, it ought not to be done too much.

c. Scating in a circular line, described by both feet. The commencement of this movement, is precisely the same as in the preceding exercise *b*; but then the toes are removed a little from the straight line, and the feet, of course, describe a circular line, the centre of which is opposite the front of the gymnick.

d. Scating with stepping over. In the midst of the course, the gymnick puts the left foot, which has given the push, over the right upon the ice, the right being raised, and the motion being continued on the left. If this *stepping over*, or changing the feet, is continued, the course turns into a circular line, either to the right, or left side.

Scating cannot form a part of the regular instruction in gymnasticks, like the rest of the exercises described, both on account of the place requisite for practising it, and its requiring personal practice, continued for a considerable time, rather than much advice or direction; yet it serves to increase the strength and dexterity to such a degree, that it would be wrong to omit it here, though it cannot belong to those exercises, practised in a common gymnasium.

VII. EXERCISES ON THE SINGLE BAR.

Instruments:

1. The *single bar* (see pl. VII, fig. K.), is a round pole, 2 1-4, or 2 1-2 inches thick, resting upon posts (see pl. VII, fig. L). The distance from one post to another must exceed the length of a person. For beginners the bar must be as high as their shoulders, or crown of the head; for those more practised, so high as to oblige them to spring in order to take hold.

The ground, below the bar, must be soft.

2. The *sliding bar*, consists of a piece of wood, 16 feet long, 6 inches thick, on the lower part 3, on the upper part 2 inches broad, rounded on the upper part, and resting on two posts, one of which is six, the other eight feet, above ground.

All exercises performed on the *single bar*, may be comprised in two classes:

A. Exercises in hanging.
B. Exercises with swinging.

EXPLANATIONS.

I. All *hanging* on the single bar, is either:

a. *side-hanging*, when the line of the shoulders is parallel with the bar (see pl. V, fig. 3), or

b. *cross-hanging*, when the line of the shoulders cuts the bar at right angles. See pl. V, fig. 1.

II. The *grasp* on the single bar, is:

a. in *side-hanging*:

1. *from above*, when the hands, or arms, are placed above upon the bar, the thumbs inwards. See pl. V, fig. 3, 4, and 5.

2. *from beneath*, when the hands, or arms, passing through below the bar, are placed upon the bar, the thumbs outwards. See pl. V, fig. 6.

3. *double grasp*, when one hand is placed from above, the thumb inwards, the other from beneath, the thumb outwards. See pl. V, fig. 7.

b. in *cross-hanging*, there is only *one* grasp, one hand, or one arm, always taking hold on each side. See pl. V, fig. 1, and 2.

III. *Upon* the bar, the pupil can be in the following situations:

a. *Sitting*:

1. *side-seat*, upon both thighs, (see pl. VII, fig. 1),
2. *riding-seat*,

upon one thigh, the other leg hanging down, behind the bar, the line of the shoulders being parallel with the bar, (see pl. IV, fig. 2);

upon neither thigh, the face turned along the bar, one leg on each side.

b. Resting:

a. belly on, or above the bar, legs closed on one side, hands with the side-grasp, before the body. See pl. IV, fig. 3 ;

b. the arms behind the body, the back against the bar.

c. Being suspended, when the body, supported by the hands, does not touch the bar ; this may be done :

1. from the position of *sitting*,
    side-seat (see pl. IV, fig. 1),
    riding seat
        upon one thigh (see pl. IV, fig. 2),
        upon neither thigh ;
2. from the position of *resting*,
    the arms before the body (see pl. IV, fig. 4),
    the arms behind the body.

A. EXERCISES IN HANGING.

I. *Hanging on :* any hanging on the bar, with hands, or arms, in upright position.

a. Hands, or arms, before the body :

1. *cross-hanging*
    with the hands (see pl. V, fig. 1), the arms being either
        stretched, or
        bent,
    with the lower part of the arms. See pl. V, fig. 2.
2. *side-hanging :*
    a. grasping from above,
        with the hands (see pl. V, fig. 3), the arms being either

stretched, or
bent,
with the lower part of the arms, (see pl. V, fig. 4),
with the upper part of the arms, (see pl. V, fig. 5);
b. *grasping from beneath:*
with the hands (see pl. V, fig. 6), the arms being either
stretched, or
bent;
c. *grasping from either side:*
with the hands (see pl. V, fig. 7), the arms being either
stretched, or
bent.
b. *Hands, or arms, behind the body;*
only *side-hanging;*
1. *grasping from above*
with the hands (see pl. V, fig. 8),
with the lower part of the arms (see pl. V, fig. 9);
2. *grasping from beneath:*
with the hands (see pl. V. fig. 10);
3. *grasping from either side:*
with the hands (see pl. V, fig. 11).

It is well to practise these different kinds of *hanging on* with a view to duration. In order to ascertain the comparative strength of a number of gymnicks, these, as many as find room, may occupy the sliding bar.

II. *Hanging close to the bar*, when the gymnick, from one of the preceding positions (page 59 and 60, I), throws his legs up to the bar; the swing, necessary for doing this, is called *swinging to.*

a. *Arms before the body:*
1. from the *cross-hanging* (see pl. V, fig. 1; page 59, I, a. 1), the feet are thrown up to the bar, (see pl. IV. fig. 9);

2. from the *side-hanging*.

grasping from above (see pl. V, fig. 3, and pl. IV, fig. 10, page 59, I, a, 2, a),

grasping from beneath (see pl. V, fig. 6, page 60, I, a, 2, b),

grasping from either side (see pl. V, fig. 7; page 60, I, a, 2, c).

The toes and knees come to rest between the hands. See pl. IV, fig. 10; or

the legs are thrown over the bar, from above, so that the knees come to rest upon the bar, the hands between them.

b. *Arms behind the body:*

from the *side-hanging*

grasping from above (see pl. V, fig. 8, page 60, I, b, 1),

grasping from beneath (see pl. V, fig. 10; page 60, I, b, 2),

grasping from either side (see pl. V, fig. 11; page 60, I, b, 3).

The knees come to rest between the hands.

We think it unnecessary to enumerate all the mixed exercises of *hanging close to the bar*, because they may easily be found; as:

hanging with one hand, and one arm,

with one hand, *or* one arm; then

hanging on one leg,

and the different kinds of *hanging close to the bar*, arising from these kinds of hanging.

Two other exercises will be mentioned which are not *hanging close to the bar*, as described in II, (page 60), yet resemble it.

1. The gymnick takes hold from the side, grasping from above, throws up his legs, so that his toes come to rest against the bar, between the hands, and the knees between the arms, as in the position described II, a, 2,

(see page 61, and pl. IV, fig. 10); the toes being firmly pressed to the bar, the body passes through between the arms, the back is drawn in, and bent, the head turned to the opposite side, and raised.

2. The gymnick, in the position of cross-hanging, throws his legs up to the bar, as in the position described II, a, 1 (see page 60, and pl. IV, fig. 9); the body is entirely turned, so that the belly is towards the ground. The top of one foot is placed upon the bar, the other on the heel of the former. Hands and arms are likewise turned. This exercise may be performed with one arm, and foot.

III. *Hanging in a suspended position*, when the pupil raises his legs from one of the positions, described under I and II, so far above the bar as to come in a suspended situation, that is to say, to rest quietly, without touching the bar with any part of the body, except the hands.

This exercise is to be performed, at first,
>from the ground, then
without starting from the ground.

a. *Hands before the body:*
1. *cross-hanging*, the legs separate (see pl. IV, fig. 11);
2. *side-hanging*, the legs are closed,
grasping from above,
grasping from beneath,
grasping from either side.

b. *Hands behind the body:*
only *side-hanging;*
grasping from above,
grasping from beneath,
grasping from either side.

In performing the exercise, III, *b*, the back must be drawn in, the head is below, the legs above the bar.

IV. *Hanging down;* any position, in which the pupil

hangs down from the bar, on his feet, or lower part of the legs, the head turned downwards.

   a. Cross-hanging, on the feet; the feet are crossed, and the toes twisted. See pl. IV, fig. 5.

   b. Side-hanging:

     1. on the knees (see pl. IV, fig. 6),
        on both,
        on one, alternately; on each knee so long, as is necessary to see, whether the pupil is able to bear his weight;
     2. on the toes (see pl. IV, fig. 7),
     3. on the heels (see pl. IV, fig. 8).

The two last kinds are to be practised on a bar, where the pupil's head almost touches the ground, lest it should suffer by a fall.

V. *Moving in hanging*, in the positions described above, Exerc. I, (page 59 and 60,) III, *a*, 1 and 2, (page 62), and IV, *b*, 1, (page 63). This exercise is an important means for strengthening the arms, shoulders, breast, and belly; it must be practised for some time.

Instrument:

The common *bar* may be used for this exercise, but it is better to have a particular instrument. This should be a quadrilateral or hexagonal stand of bars joined (see pl. VII, fig. M), on the inside of which the motion should be continued, as long as the strength allows.

Hanging on one hand, and arm, is to be exercised as the best preparatory exercise for *moving along*.

Each hand must be able to cling to the bar, until the hand of the other arm, stretched out, has touched the thigh. The longer this hanging on one hand is continued, the more difficult it is. It may be practised

   a. on the hand
     cross-hanging,
     side-hanging
        from above, and

from beneath.

b. on the lower part of the arm, or *elbow*.

c. on the upper part of the arm, or *shoulder*.

The two last kinds only in side-hanging.

Moving along may be practised:

a. in all kinds of *hanging on*, described under Exerc. I, (page 59, and 60);

b. in all kinds of *hanging close to the bar*, described under Exerc. II, (page 60, and 61);

c. in all kinds of *hanging in a suspended position*, described under Exerc. III, (page 62);

d. in *hanging on the knees*, described under Exerc. IV, *b*, 1, (page 63, pl. IV, fig. 6);

e. changing and *turning the grasp:*

1. *changing the grasp*, when the pupil remains on one side of the bar, and makes half revolutions around his axis. By the revolution of the body, and the changing of the hands, the latter come from the grasp from above into that from beneath, and the reverse;

2. *turning the grasp*, only backwards, when the pupil is in the position of cross-hanging, the hands turned so, that the thumbs stand upwards.

The gymnick accomplishes the posture, just described, in the following manner. He is standing below the bar, as if to take hold for *cross-hanging*, but instead of doing this, the right hand passes beneath the bar, and takes hold from the left side, and the left hand, passing beneath the bar, from the right.

In all kinds of *moving in a hanging position*, the legs must be stretched, and closed, unless a particular posture of them be made a part of the exercise.

VI. *Raising the body*, from most of the positions described under Exerc. I, (page 59, and 60), as high as possible, by mere drawing, without the elbows forming a horizontal line; it must be considerably practised, for, without some dexterity in it, no exercise, without starting from the ground, can be performed.

a. Cross-hanging: (see Exerc. I, *a*, 1, page 59, pl. V, fig. 1); so far that the shoulders, right and left by turns, touch the bar.

b. Side-hanging:

grasping from beneath (see Exerc. I, *a*, 2, *b*, page 60; pl. V, fig. 6),

grasping from above (see Exerc. I. *a*, 2, a, page 59; pl. V, fig. 3),

grasping from either side (see Exerc. I, *a*, 2, *c*, page 60; pl. V, fig. 7);

so high, that the eyes, mouth, or chin, reach over the bar.

The body can be, during this exercise,

1. stretched;
2. bent in the knees;
3. bent in the knees, and hips;
4. bent in the hips alone, which is, by far, the most difficult.

Hanging on one hand, the arm bent, and letting down slowly, is the best preparatory exercise for *raising the body with one arm*, which is one of the most difficult exercises.

VII. *Changing the grasp.* The exercise VI, *Raising the body*, must precede this, being preparatory for it. The body is raised high enough to gain time for changing the grasp;

a. from the grasp from above (see Expl. II, *a*, 1, page 58; pl. V, fig. 3) to that from beneath (see Expl. II, *a*, 2, page 58; pl. V, fig. 6), and the reverse;

b. from either side (see Expl. II, *a*, 3, page 58; pl. V, fig. 7);

c. from hanging on the elbows from above (see Expl. II, *a*, 3, page 58; pl. V. fig. 4) to the grasp from beneath (see Expl. II, *a*, 2, page 58; pl. V, fig. 6), and the reverse;

d. with one hand. The gymnick draws himself up, and remains hanging on his right hand, the arm bent, then loosens his grasp, and, with the same hand, takes hold of the bar from the opposite side. The same is to be practised with the left hand.

VIII. *Transition from the position of hanging on, side-hanging* (see Expl. I, *a*, page 58; pl. V, fig. 3) *to the position of resting on the bar* (see Expl. III, *b*. 1, page 59; pl. IV, fig. 3). The arms are bent, elbows raised above the bar, and then stretched;

    a. placing the lower part of the arms upon the bar ;

    b. raising the elbows one after the other ;

    c. raising the elbows at a time.

IX. *Moving the body, resting on, or suspended by, the arms ;*

    a. the *body resting* on the arms,

    1. the arms before the body (see Expl. III, *b*. 1, page 59 ; pl. IV, fig. 3),

        to the right, and

        to the left ;

    2. the arms behind the body (see Expl. IV, *b*. 2, page 59),

        to the right, and

        to the left ;

    b. the *body being suspended,*

    1. in the side-seat (see Expl. III, *a*. 1, page 58 ; pl. IV, fig. 1),

        to the right, and

        to the left ;

    2. in the riding-seat,

      a. one thigh above the bar, (see Expl. III, *a*, 2, page 59 ; pl. IV, fig. 2),

        to the right, and

        to the left ;

      b. one thigh on either side, (see Expl. III, *a*, 2, page 59),

        to the right, and

        to the left.

Both kinds of this exercise (*a* and *b*), may be performed with
> *one hand after the other*, or
> with *both at a time*.

X. *Lowering*, and *raising*;
  a. resting:
    1. the arms, before the body (see Expl. III, *b*. 1, page 59; pl. IV, fig. 3), bend gradually so low that the mouth touches the bar;
    2. the arms, behind the body (see Expl. III, *b*, 2, page 59), bend gradually so low that the lower part of the shoulders touches the bar;
  b. being suspended:
    1. in the riding-seat,
      upon one thigh (see Expl. III, *c*. 1, page 59; pl. IV, fig. 2);
      on neither thigh; in raising, the legs must straddle, in lowering, the elbows bend;
    2. the body on one side (see Expl. III, *c*. 2, page 59; pl. IV, fig. 4).

B. EXERCISES WITH SWINGING.
Preparatory Exercises.

Since the exercises, performed with swinging, frequently carry the gymnick upon the bar, so as to sit upon it, it is well for him to obtain some firmness in this position. The following exercises will enable him to attain that object.

I. *Sitting.*
  a. Side-seat, upon both thighs (see Expl. III, *a*, 1, page 58; pl. IV, fig. 1);
    taking hold with both hands,
      grasping from above,
      grasping from beneath;
    taking hold with one hand, alternately,
      grasping from above,
      grasping from beneath;
    not taking hold at all.

b. Riding-seat, upon one thigh (see Expl. III, a, 2, page 59; pl. IV, fig. 2), alternately;
  taking hold with both hands,
    grasping from above,
    grasping from beneath;
  taking hold with one hand, alternately,
    grasping from above,
    grasping from beneath;
  not taking hold at all.

c. Riding-seat, upon neither thigh (see Expl. III, a, 2, page 59);
  taking hold with both hands, from either side,
    hands before the body,
    hands behind the body;
  taking hold with one hand,
    hand before the body,
    hand behind the body;
  not taking hold at all.

II. *Changing the seat.*

a. From the position of *side-seat, upon both thighs*, into that of *riding-seat, upon neither thigh.* The gymnick raises his right leg, and passes it over the bar, the right hand being lifted. The same is to be done with the left leg.

b. From the position of *riding-seat, upon neither thigh*, into that of *side-seat, upon both thighs.* The gymnick raises his right leg, and passes it over the bar, the right hand being lifted. The same is to be done with the left leg.

These two *changes of seat* may be practised:
  taking hold with both hands, the right hand being lifted, when the right leg passes over the bar, and the reverse;
  taking hold with one hand,
    behind the body, the left hand, if the right leg moves, and the reverse;

before the body, the right hand, if the right leg passes, the hand being lifted, whilst the leg passes over the bar;

not taking hold at all.

These two *changes of seat* are to be combined in this way:

from *side-seat, upon both thighs*, to *riding-seat, upon neither thigh*, with the right leg;

from *riding-seat, upon neither thigh*, to *side-seat, upon both thighs*, with the left leg;

from *side-seat, upon both thighs*, to *riding-seat, upon neither thigh*, with the left leg;

from *riding-seat, upon neither thigh*, to *side-seat, upon both thighs*, with the right leg.

The same combination is to be gone through, beginning with the left leg.

c. From the position of *side-seat, upon both thighs*, on *one* side of the bar, to the same on the *other*. The gymnick, turning a little to the right, raises both his legs closed towards the right, and passes them to the other side;

taking hold with one hand, that is to say, exchanging the grasp with the left hand, while the legs pass over the bar, for that with the right hand;

not taking hold at all; the upper part of the body is principally to be used for preserving the equilibrium.

The same is to be practised left, and, after some practice, to be continued, right and left, alternately.

Exercises.

There are *three* kinds of *swinging*:

I. *Swinging up*, the motion which carries the pupil upon the bar from either of the following positions,

a. *Hanging close to the bar* (see Exerc. A, II, page 60);

b. Hanging in a suspended position (see Exerc. A, III, page 62);

c. Hanging down (see Exerc. A, IV, page 62).

II. *Swinging around*, any revolution of the pupil around the axis of the bar.

III. *Swinging off*, any motion which carries the pupil from the position of *resting* (see Expl. III, *b*, page 59; pl. IV, fig. 3), or of *side-seat* (see Expl. III, *a*, 1, page 58; pl. IV, fig. 1.), forwards or backwards, to the ground, with at least half a revolution around his axis.

No regular *swinging off*, therefore, can be performed from the *riding-seat*, on one thigh, or when one leg is on either side (see Expl. III, *a*, 2).

Every *swinging up* is preceded by a *swinging to*, which is necessary in some exercises, already described, viz.

Hanging close to the bar (see Exerc. A, II, page 60, with the two exercises described page 61, & 62, 1 and 2),

Hanging in a suspended position (see Exerc. A, III, page 62),

Hanging down (see Exerc. A, IV, page 62).

Swinging to can be performed

from the ground, or

from hanging,

the latter of which is more difficult.

I. SWINGING UP.

First kind:

whereby the gymnick comes to sit in the *riding-seat, upon one thigh* (see Expl. III, *a*, 2, page 59; pl. IV, fig. 2), is performed from the following position. The hands take hold from the side, and one leg is thrown over the bar, so as to come to rest between the hands (see Exerc. A, II, *a*, 2, page 61), the other leg, hanging down, gives the swing.

It is rendered more easy, to beginners, to make the motion from the following position. The gymnick makes the *cross-hanging close to the bar* (see Exerc. A. II. *a*, 1, page

60; pl. IV, fig. 9), and then, changing the grasp from beneath, of the left hand, into that from above, with the upper part of the left arm, and sinking the left leg, swings up; or the reverse, with the right arm, and leg.

This *swinging up* can be varied so that the upper arms, lower arms, hands, one or both, rest upon the bar, on the right or left side, close together, or separated by the hanging leg, with the grasp from above, beneath, or either side. Thus a hundred and thirty-two different kinds of *swinging up*, are possible, about one half of which can be performed forwards, and backwards. Each of them is called *common swinging up*.

Two more kinds of *swinging up*, not comprised among those, described in the preceding paragraph, should be mentioned here:

   a. with arms crossed;
   b. with taking hold of the knee, beneath the bar.

Second kind:

whereby the gymnick comes to sit in the *side-seat, upon both thighs* (see Expl. III, *a*, 1, page 58; pl. IV, fig. 1); it is performed from the position of *hanging close to the bar, the arms behind the body* (see Exerc. A, II, *b*, page 61), forwards, and backwards.

The hands may take hold from above (compare pl. V, fig. 8), from beneath (compare pl. V, fig. 10), or from either side (compare pl. V, fig. 11).

The thighs may be separated by one, or both hands.

In this kind of *swinging up*, the feet may be taken hold of, instead of the bar.

Third kind:

whereby the gymnick comes to sit in the *riding-seat, one leg on each side* (see Expl. III, *a*, 2, page 59). This kind of *swinging up* is performed from *hanging in a suspended position, cross-hanging* (see Exerc. A, III, *a*, 1, page 62; pl. IV, fig. 11), right, and left.

To perform this kind of *swinging up* with more facility,

and quickness, the gymnick may take hold of the bar from the side, with both his hands from above (see Exerc. A, I, *a*, 2, *a*, page 59; pl. V, fig. 3), swing his legs up, on the other side of the bar, as if to come into the position of *hanging in a suspended position, side-hanging* (see Exerc. A, III, *a*, 2, page 62), and passes, throwing back one leg, below the bar, through the position of *hanging in a suspended position, cross-hanging* (see Exerc. A, III, *a*, 1, page 62; pl. IV, fig. 11).

Fourth kind:

whereby the gymnick comes to *rest* on his arms (see Expl. III, *b*, 1, page 59; pl. IV, fig. 3); it is performed from *hanging in a suspended position, side-hanging* (see Exerc. *A*, III, *a*, 2, and *b*, page 62).

a. From hanging in a suspended position, side-hanging, the arms before the body (see Exerc. *A*, III, *a*, 2, page 62):

1. *forwards*, with the head foremost; the gymnick takes hold from the side, the legs are thrown up into the position of *hanging in a suspended position* (see Exerc. *A*, III, *a*, 2, page 62), but return immediately with a strong swing, the arms draw the body up towards the bar, and bear up, so as to come to *rest* (see Expl. III, *b*, 1, page 59; pl. IV, fig. 3);

2. *backwards*, with the feet foremost; the gymnick takes hold from the side, the legs are thrown up, through the position of *hanging in a suspended position* (see Exerc. *A*, III, *a*, 2, page 62), over the bar, so that the belly comes to *rest* upon the bar (see Expl. III, *b*, 1, page 59; pl. IV, fig. 3).

b. From hanging in a suspended position, side-hanging, the arms behind the body (see Exerc. *A*, III, *b*, page 62). From this position the swinging up, can be performed only backwards, the feet foremost. The swing carries the gymnick only with the back upon the bar; the raising of the head follows, and brings him into the *rest,* the hands behind the body (see Expl. III, *b.* 2, page 59).

The movement mentioned last *(b),* as well as the preceding *(a,* 2), if performed by drawing alone, without any swinging, is much more difficult.

Fifth kind:

whereby the gymnick comes to sit in the *side-seat, upon both thighs* (see Expl. III, *a,* 1, page 58; pl. IV, fig. 1); it is performed from the position of *hanging down, sidehanging, on the knees* (see Exerc. *A,* IV, *b,* 1, page 63; pl. IV, fig. 6), forwards, and backwards, without the assistance of the hands. The arms are stretched downwards, and, thus, serve to increase the swing.

II. SWINGING AROUND.

a. Every *swinging up,* from the position of *hanging close to the bar* (see Exerc. *A,* II, page 60), or *hanging down* (see Exerc. *A,* IV, page 62), if continued, so that it carries the gymnick once, or several times, around the bar, is *one* kind of *swinging around.*

1. The *first kind of swinging up* (page 70), continued. The gymnick takes hold from the side (see Exerc. *A,* II, *a,* 2, page 61), one leg is thrown over the bar, so that it comes to rest between the hands, the other leg, hanging down, gives the swing. When the swing has carried the gymnick upon the bar (so far like the *first kind of swinging up),* he does not stop, but continues the movement, so that he swings once, or several times, around the bar. It is performed

 forwards, and

 backwards.

2. The *first kind of swinging up* (page 70) *with taking hold of the knee* beneath the bar, instead of the bar, continued. The gymnick takes hold from the side (see Exerc. *A,* II, *a,* 2, page 61), one leg is thrown over the bar, so that it comes to rest between the hands: the

hands, instead of retaining the hold of the bar, pass beneath the bar, and, locked, take hold of the knee; the other leg, hanging down, gives the swing. The motion is not stopped, when the gymnick has come to sit upon the bar, but continued once, or several times, around the bar. It is performed
> forwards, and
> backwards.

3. The *second king of swinging up* (page 71) continued. The gymnick, in the position of *hanging close to the bar, the arms behind the body* (see Exerc. *A*, II, *b*, page 61), swings himself up, so as to come to sit in the *side-seat, upon both thighs* (see Expl. III, *a*, 1, page 58; pl. IV, fig. 1); but instead of stopping there, he continues the movement, so that he is carried around the bar, once or several times. It is performed
> forwards, and
> backwards.

4. The *second kind of swinging up* (page 71) *with taking hold of the feet,* instead of the bar, continued. The gymnick, in the position of *hanging close to the bar, the arms behind the body* (see Exerc. *A*, II, *b*, page 61), swings himself up, so as to come to sit in the *side-seat, upon both thighs* (see Expl. III, *a*, 1, page 58; pl. IV, fig. 1); the hands, instead of retaining the hold of the bar, pass, from behind, below the bar, and take hold of the feet, and, then, the gymnick continues the movement, so as to swing, once or several times, around the bar. It is performed
> forwards, and
> backwards.

5. The *fifth kind of swinging up* (page 73), continued. The gymnick, in the position of *hanging down, side-hanging, in the knees* (see Exerc. *A*, IV, *b*, 1, page 63; pl. IV, fig. 6), swings himself up, without the assistance of the hands, so that he comes to sit in the *side-seat, upon*

both thighs (see Expl. III, *a*, 1, page 58; pl. IV, fig. 1); but, without stopping, he continues the movement, so that he is carried, once or several times, around the bar. Much depends upon employing the arms for improving, and regulating the swing.

In order to perform this kind of *swinging around*, it is necessary to perform, with certainty, the *swinging off*, described afterwards under III, *a*, 5.

6. The *third kind of swinging up* (page 71), continued. The gymnick, *hanging in a suspended position, cross-hanging* (see Exerc. *A*, III, *a*, 1, page 62; pl. IV, fig. 11), swings up, so that he comes to sit in the *riding-seat, one leg on each side* (see Expl. III, *a*, 2, page 59); without stopping, he continues the movement, so that he is carried, once or several times, around the bar. It is performed

to the right, and
to the left.

b. Another kind of *swinging around*, is from the position of *resting, the arms before the body* (see Expl. III, *b*, 1, page 59; pl. IV, fig. 3). It is the *fourth kind of swinging up*, from *hanging in a suspended position, side-hanging, the arms before the body* (see Exerc. *A*, III, *a*, 2, page 62), continued. It is performed

forwards, *fourth kind of swinging up, a*, 1, (page 52), continued;

backwards, *fourth kind of swinging up, a*, 2, (page 72), continued.

The belly must remain, during the movement, as close to the bar as possible.

c. A *third* kind of *swinging around*, similar to the preceding exercise *(b)*, with this difference that the hands do not take hold of the bar, but of the thighs. The gymnick, in the position of *resting, the arms before the body* (see Expl. III, *b*, 1, page 59; pl. IV, fig. 3), leans on his belly, the hands take hold of the thighs, the bar between the arms and body.

d. A fourth kind of *swinging around.* The gymnick, in the position of *hanging on, arms behind the body, grasping from above, with the lower part of the arms* (see Exerc. *A,* I, *b,* 1, page 60 ; pl. V, fig. 9), swings, once or several times, around the bar. It is performed
    forwards, and
    backwards.

e. A *fifth* kind of *swinging around.* The gymnick, in the position of *hanging on, arms before the body, side-hanging, grasping from above, with the upper part of the arms* (see Exerc. *A,* I, *a,* 2, ä, page 59 ; pl. V, fig. 5), swings, once or several times, around the bar, the feet foremost.

f. A *sixth* kind of *swinging around.* The gymnick takes hold from the side (see Expl. II, *a,* page 58 ; pl. V, fig. 3, 6, or 7), forces his legs up, on the other side of the bar, and swings over (so far it is like the *fourth kind of swinging up, a,* 2, page 72) ; but instead of coming to rest upon the belly, he continues the movement, so that he, without having touched the bar at all, descends on the same spot, whence he started.

III. SWINGING OFF.

All kinds of *swinging off,* must be performed with feet and legs closed.

a. Swinging off, the gymnick making an *entire revolution* around his axis.

    1. Forwards, from the position of resting. The gymnick, in the position of *resting, the arms before the body* (see Expl. III, *b,* 1, page 59 ; pl. IV, fig. 3), turns over, head foremost. Beginners may grasp from beneath, or with thumbs outwards (see pl. V, fig. 6) ; but it may be done as well, grasping from above, or with thumbs inwards (see pl. V, fig. 3) although it has the appearance of not affording perfect security ; it depends upon this, that the hands follow the movement of the body.

A variation of the same exercise is, to raise the back part of the body (in a manner, similar to raising, the seventh preparatory exercise for vaulting, (page 22, VII; pl. III, fig. 4), before turning over.

2. Forwards, with placing the knees on the bar. The gymnick, in the position of *resting, the arms before the body* (see Expl. III, *b*, 1, page 59; pl. IV, fig. 3), draws up his back, till the knees have reached the top of, and rest on, the bar, then turns over, head foremost.

3. Backwards, from the side-seat. The gymnick, in the position of *side-seat, upon both thighs* (see Expl. III, *a*, 1, page 58; pl. IV, fig. 1), turns over backwards. The hands may grasp from above, beneath, or either side; the first grasp is the safest for beginners.

4. Backwards, from the side-seat. The gymnick, in the position of *side-seat, upon both thighs* (see Expl. III, *a*, 1, page 58; pl. IV, fig. 1), takes hold of his feet, the arms behind the body, which hold, however, is loosened again, after öne half of the revolution is accomplished.

5. Backwards, from the side-seat. The gymnick, in the position of *side-seat, upon both thighs* (see Expl. III, *a*, 1, page 58; pl. IV, fig. 1), throws himself, without using the hands for holding, backwards, into the position of *hanging down, side-hanging, on the knees* (see Exerc. *A*, IV, *b*, 1, page 63; pl. IV, fig. 6), advances, by means of the same swing, on the other side, so far, that his body is in a horizontal line, looses the hold of his knees, and comes to stand before the bar.

This kind of swinging off, must, at first, be practised from the position of *hanging down, side-hanging, on the knees* (see Exerc. *A*, IV, *b*, 1, page 63; pl. IV, fig. 6); then the sinking slowly from the position of *side-seat, upon both thighs,* into that of *hanging-down, side-hanging, on the knees;* at last both movements, together, are to be practised, but with great caution, and, in the beginning, with assistance.

b. Swinging off, the gymnick making *half a revolution* around his axis, after which a second, in opposite direction, follows.

1. *Forwards, from the side-seat.* The gymnick, in the position of *side-seat, upon both thighs* (see Expl. III, *a*, 1, page 58; pl. IV, fig. 1), turns over, forwards; when he has revolved half around the bar, so that his head is below it, (that is to say, in the position of *hanging down, side-hanging, on the knees*) the knees loosen their hold, the legs sink down, and the gymnick comes to stand before the bar.

This kind of *swinging off*, may be varied in this way, that the gymnick, in the position of *side-seat, upon both thighs*, raises himself on his arms (see Expl. III, *c*, 1, page 59), brings both hands together, so that they touch, and swings off.

2. *Forwards, from the side-seat.* The gymnick, in the position of *side-seat, upon both thighs* (see Expl. III, *a*, 1, page 58; pl. IV, fig. 1), takes hold of his feet, the arms behind the bar, turns over, forwards; when he has revolved half around the bar, the hands loosen their hold, then the knees likewise, the legs sink down, and the gymnick comes to stand before the bar.

Both these kinds of *swinging off*, (*b*, 1 and 2), the gymnick making *half a revolution* around his axis, are changed into *swinging off*, the gymnick making an *entire revolution* around his axis, if the second part of the following exercise (IV, *b*) is added.

IV. SWINGING THROUGH.

Swinging through is a kind of *swinging around*, the axis of which is not the bar, but the shoulders of the gymnick.

a. Forwards. The gymnick takes hold from the side, forces up his legs on the other side, as if to perform the *hanging close to the bar, arms before the body, side-hanging, the toes and knees between the hands* (see Exerc. *A*, II, *a*, 2, page 61; pl. IV, fig. 10), draws on the toes, and passes through between the arms; after the legs have passed through between the arms, the body is stretched downwards, as much as possible. See pl. V, fig. 8.

b. Backwards. From this position, just described, the gymnick returns, drawing up his back, and passing through between his arms, so as to come into the first position.

This exercise should be repeated several times, forwards and backwards, without touching the ground, either at the commencement, or end of the movement.

V. SWINGING UNDER.

The gymnick takes hold from the side, and forces his legs up, on the other side, almost so high, as to reach the position of *hanging in a suspended position, arms before the body, side-hanging* (see Exerc. *A*, III, *a*, 2, page 62), but then the whole body follows this movement, and, the back being drawn in, is forced, in a high and long arch, to the ground, standing. The hands should not cling to the bar too long, nor leave it too soon.

VI. SWINGING FORWARDS AND BACKWARDS.

The gymnick takes hold from the side, from above, or with thumbs inward, and swings, arms, body, and legs being perfectly straight, forwards and backwards. The moment the motion backwards changes into that of forwards, the hands renew their grasp, and thus the swinging is continued for some time.

In loosening the grasp, or in alighting, care must be taken to do it at the proper time. The most convenient time is, when the hands are about to renew their grasp. Another mode, like the latter part of the preceding exercise, *swinging under*, is, before the motion forwards changes into that of backwards, to force the body up, the back being considerably drawn in, and to alight in a high, and long arch.

The *exercises of the single bar*, have been enumerated, and described according to their natural arrangement, as they are derived from, and belong to, one another. But in practising, in these exercises, as well as in all others, an arrangement according to their greater facility or difficulty, should be pursued. This, indeed, must be left to the judgment of the instructor, who will make alterations according to the natural dexterity of the gymnicks; but we propose the following series of these exercises, which, we think, will be suitable for most cases.

I. Position of *hanging on, arms before the body, side-hanging, grasping from above, with the hands* (see Exerc. *A*, I, *a*, 2, a, page 59; pl. V, fig. 3).

    Moving in this position (see Exerc. *A*, V, page 64)
        to the right,
        to the left.

II. Position of *hanging on, arms before the body, side-hanging, grasping from above, with the lower parts of the arms* (see Exerc. *A*, I, *a*, 2, a, page 60; pl. V, fig. 4).

    Moving in this position (see Exerc. *A*, V, page 64)
        to the right,
        to the left.

III. Position of *hanging on, arms before the body, side-hanging, grasping from above, with the upper parts of the arms* (see Exerc. *A*, I, *a*, 2, a, page 60; pl. V, fig. 5).

    Moving in this position (see Exerc. *A*, V, page 64)
        to the right,
        to the left.

IV. Position of *hanging on, arms before the body, cross-hanging, with the hands* (see Exerc. *A*, I, *a*, 1, page 59; pl. V, fig. 1).

    Moving in this position (see Exerc. *A*, V, page 64)
        forwards,
        backwards.

V. *Raising the body* (see Exerc. *A*, VI, page 64), as often as possible,

    a. cross-hanging (see Exerc. *A*, VI, *a*, page 65);

    b. side-hanging, grasping from above (see Exerc. *A*, VI, *b*, page 65).

VI. Position of *hanging close to the bar, arms before the body, cross-hanging* (see Exerc. *A*, II, *a*, 1, page 60; pl. IV, fig. 9).

It should be repeated three, or more, times, that is to say, the swinging up, which produces that position, is to be repeated so often.

VII. Position of *hanging close to the bar, arms before the body, side-hanging, grasping from above, the toes and knees between the hands* (see Exerc. *A*, II, *a*, 2, page 61; pl. IV, fig. 10).

It should be repeated three, or more times, that is to say, the swinging up, which produces that position, is to be repeated so often.

VIII. Position of *hanging down, side-hanging, on the knees* (see Exerc. *A*, IV, *b*, 1, page 63; pl. IV, fig. 6).

a. on both knees,
b. on one knee, by turns.

IX. *Hanging in a suspended position, arms before the body, cross-hanging* (see Exerc. *A*, III, *a*, 1, page 62; pl. IV, fig. 11). It is to be repeated three times, and the gymnick should, each time, continue it so long, as is necessary to see, whether he is able to remain, in this position, for some time.

X. *Hanging in a suspended position, arms before the body, side-hanging* (see Exerc. *A*, III, *a*, 2, page 62). It is to be repeated three times, and the gymnick should, each time, continue it so long, as is necessary to see, whether he is able to remain, for some time, in this position.

XI. *Swinging up, first kind, with the left knee* (see Exerc. *B*, I, first kind, page 70); after this the left leg is brought back behind the bar; then *swinging off, forwards, from the position of resting* (see Exerc. *B*, III, *a*, 1, page 76).

XII. *Swinging up, first kind, with the right knee* (see Exerc. *B*, I, first kind, page 70); after this the left leg is brought forwards, so that the gymnick comes to sit in the side-seat, upon both thighs; then *swinging off, backwards, from the side-seat* (see Exerc. *B*, III, *a*, 3, page 77).

XIII. *Swinging up, fourth kind, the arms before the body, backwards* (see Exerc. *B*, I, fourth kind, *a*, 2, page 72); then *swinging off, forwards, from the position of resting* (see Exerc. *B*, III, *a*, 1, page 76).

XIV. *Lowering, and raising, in the position of resting, the arms before the body* (see Exerc. *A*, X, *a*, 1, page 67).

XV. *Transition from the position of hanging on, side-hanging, to the position of resting upon the bar* (see Exerc. *A*, VIII, page 66).

XVI. *Swinging up, fourth kind, the arms before the body, forwards* (see Exerc. *B*, I, fourth kind, *a*, 1, page 72), and *swinging off, forwards, from the position of resting* (see Exerc. *B*, III, *a*, 1, page 76).

XVII. *Moving, the body resting on the arms, the arms before the body* (see Exerc. *A*, IX, *a*, 1, page 66), to the right, and left.

XVIII. *Swinging through* (see Exerc. *B*, IV, *a*, page 78); then *swinging up, fourth kind, the arms behind the body* (see Exerc. *B*, I, fourth kind, *b*, page 72); then *swinging off, backwards, from the side-seat, upon both thighs* (see Exerc. *B*, III, *a*, 3, page 77).

XIX. *Raising the body, cross-hanging* (see Exerc. *A*, VI, *a*, page 65), repeated as often as possible.

XX. *Swinging up, second kind* (see Exerc. *B*, I, second kind, page 71), forwards and backwards; then any kind of *swinging off* (see Exerc. *B*, III, page 76).

XXI. *Swinging up, third kind* (see Exerc. *B*, I, third kind, page 71), to the right, and left; then any kind of *swinging off* (see Exerc. *B*, III, page 76).

XXII. *First kind of swinging around* (see Exerc. *B*, II, page 73):

    a. from the *first kind of swinging up* (see Exerc. *B*, II, *a*, 1, page 73), forwards, and backwards;

    b. from the *first kind of swinging up, with taking hold*

of the knee (see Exerc. *B*, II, *a*, 2, page 73), forwards, and backwards;

  c. from the *second kind of swinging up* (see Exerc. *B*, II, *a*, 3, page 74), forwards, and backwards;

  d. from the *third kind of swinging up* (see Exerc. *B*, II, *a*, 6, page 75); to the right, and left.

XXIII. *Second king of swinging around* (see Exerc. *B*, II, *b*, page 75), forwards, and backwards.

XXIV. *Swinging up, fourth kind, the arms behind the body* (see Exerc. *B*, I, fourth kind, *b*, page 72), performed by drawing alone.

XXV. *Fifth kind of swinging around* (see Exerc. *B*, II, *e*, page 76).

XXVI. *Sixth kind of swinging around* (see Exerc. B, II, *f*, page 76).

XXVII. *Swinging through* (see Exerc. *B*, IV, page 78); forwards, and backwards.

XXVIII. *Swinging under* (see Exerc. *B*, V, page 79).

XXIX. *Swinging off, backwards, from the side-seat*, without using the hands (see Exerc. *B*, III, *a*, 5, page 77).

XXX. *Moving, with changing, and turning the grasp* (see Exerc. *A*, V, *e*, 1, and 2, page 64).

XXXI. *Changing the grasp* (see Exerc. *A*, VII, page 65).

XXXII. *Moving, the body being suspended by the arms* (see Exerc. *A*, IX, *b*, page 66).

VIII. EXERCISES ON THE PARALLEL BARS.

Instrument:

The *parallel bars* (see pl. VII, fig. H), consist of two horizontal, and parallel pieces of wood, or bars, each of which is eight feet long, and resting on two posts. Each bar is three inches thick, and 2 1-2 broad; above and at the ends rounded, and without sharp edges below. The posts may be thicker, but must be lessened, towards the bars, to the size of the bars (see pl. VII, fig. I), especially on the outside of the bars; the posts, too, must be without sharp edges; they are inserted one foot from the end of the bars.

The parallel bars must not be higher, than the arm-pit, for beginners; for those more skilled, they may reach to the crown of the head, and beyond. It is of great importance, never to try a new exercise on bars higher, than the arm-pit.

All *exercises on the parallel bars* may be arranged under two heads:

A. All *exercises with raising, resting, and bearing* up, the only object of which is to support the body by means of the arms.

B. All *exercises with swinging*, where the supporting arms are merely means for the end, and a dexterous swing, together with a regular motion of the body, the chief object.

A. EXERCISES WITH RAISING, RESTING, AND BEARING UP.

I. *Hopping.* The gymnick is standing at the end of the bars, each hand taking hold of one bar, the hands collateral with the body, not advanced, the elbows raised, and turned outwards, not backwards (see pl. II, fig. 4), hops up so high that the arms are stretched, (see pl. II, fig. 3), descends, as soon as he has reached that height, starts again, without remaining on the ground, and so on. (Compare Preparatory Exercise III, *a*, and *b*, page 2, and Preparatory Exercises for Vaulting I, page 21, and 22). This exercise may be performed

a. with bending the knees,
b. without bending the knees.

Another kind of the same exercise is, to take hold of the bars so that the thumbs are on the outside, the fingers on the inside.

Both kinds of *hopping* must be performed merely by the elastic spring of the feet, not by pulling, or bearing up with the arms. The bending, and stretching of the arms accompanies the movement, but does not produce it. Falling forwards of the upper part of the body, during the movement, is to be avoided; the whole body ought to form a perpendicular line.

If the bars reach to the crown of the head, and beyond, this exercise becomes *hopping with bearing up*.

II. *Lowering*, and *rising*. The gymnick hops up, as described in the preceding exercise, so as to rest on his arms (see plate II, fig. 3), stretched out, slowly bends, at first a little, by degrees so low, that the arm-pits approach the hands; then rises again. This exercise is to be performed

    a. the thumbs on the inside, and the fingers on the outside;

    b. the thumbs on the outside, and the fingers on the inside.

III. *Lowering*, and *touching the bars, or the hands, with the mouth*.

It is the preceding exercise (II), connected with *touching*; it should be exercised alternately, right and left; after each touch the arms must be stretched again. It is to be practised

    a. the thumbs on the inside, and the fingers on the outside, the mouth touching

        1. the bars,

        2. the hands;

    b. the thumbs on the outside, and the fingers on the inside, the mouth touching

        1. the bars,

        2. the hands.

IV. *Lowering upon the elbows*, and *rising*. The gymnick, in the middle of the bars, hops up, so as to rest on his arms (see pl. II, fig. 3), bends

    a. one arm, after the other, so as to rest with the whole lower part of the arms upon the bars, and rises again, *one* arm after the other. The last combination of this exercise is

    1. sinking with the right, with the left,
    2. rising with the right, with the left;
    3. sinking with the left, with the right,
    4. rising with the left, with the right.

b. Or the gymnick bends *both* arms at a time, and raises himself again, stretching *both* arms at a time.

V. *Raising.* The gymnick is in the position of resting on his arms (see pl. II, fig. 3), in the middle of the bars, raises both his legs, stretched, slowly

    a. forwards, when the belly is drawn in (see pl. II, fig. 5),

    b. backwards, when the back is drawn in.

The whole movement should be performed without any swing, and several times in succession, the lowering the legs being performed as slowly, as the raising. From this exercise are derived

VI. *Suspending* (See pl. II, fig. 6). When the legs are raised

    a. forwards, they are

      1. separated, and rest above the bars, in a suspended, and straddling position;

      2. moved to one side, and rest closed above *one* bar, in a suspended position

        above the right,

        above the left bar;

    b. backwards, they hang down, behind the arms,

      1. separated, over both bars, in a suspended, and straddling position,

      2. closed, over one bar, in a suspended position,

        over the right,

        over the left bar.

The body is, in neither kind, allowed to touch the arms.

VII. When the legs are raised, as described under V,

    a. forwards, they pass over one bar, and the gymnick

alights on the outside of the bars. It is to be practised
1. right, over the right bar,
2. left, over the left bar.

b. When the legs are raised backwards, they pass over one bar, and the gymnick alights on the outside of the bars. It is to be performed
1. right, over the right bar,
2. left, over the left bar.

In alighting the hand, opposite to the side on which the gymnick descends, takes hold of the bar. Compare, in general, Exerc. *B*, II, and III.

VIII. *Moving along, upon the hands.* The motion should not be produced by bending, or shaking the legs, nor drawing up the back, but by the elastic movement, or spring, of the joints of the hands. The body should be perfectly straight, and steady, during the whole movement.

a. The body resting on the hands, hanging down, the thumbs on the inside, or outside of the bars;
1. with arms stretched, (see pl. II, fig. 3),
    with one hand after the other,
    with both hands at a time;
2. with arms bent, when the elbows must be higher than the shoulders,
    with one hand after the other,
    with both hands at a time.

b. In a suspended position;
1. the legs being raised forwards (see Exerc. *A*, V, page 86; pl. II, fig. 5),
    with one hand after the other,
    with both hands at a time;
2. when raised, moved to one side, over one bar;
    with one hand after the other,
        over the right,
        over the left bar;
    with both hands at a time,
        over the right,
        over the left bar.

Sometimes this exercise is performed, the legs being separated, after they have been raised (see Exerc. *A*, VI, *a*, 1, page 86); but it is not prudent to make very great exertions, the legs being separated.

IX. *Turning*. The body, resting on the hands, (see pl. II, fig. 3), makes, by the pushing off of the hands, half a revolution around its perpendicular axis, whereby the hands exchange their places, and the face is directed to the side, where the back first was. It is at first to be practised

 a. with one hand after the other,
  1. to the right,
  2. to the left side ;
 b. then with both hands at a time,
  1. to the right,
  2. to the left side.

B. EXERCISES WITH SWINGING.

I. *Changing the seat.* The gymnick rests on his hands (see pl. II, fig. 3), in the middle of the bars, the hands keep immoveably the same hold; the legs, closed, and stretched, are thrown from one bar upon the other, or, on the same bar, from before the hands to behind them.

 a. From one bar over the other, right and left, before the hands (Compare Exerc. *B*, II, and IV);
  1. the arms stretched,
  2. the arms bent, and the elbows reaching over the shoulders,
  3. the arms bent, and the lower part of them resting on the bars.
 b. From one bar over the other, right and left, behind the hands (Compare Exerc. *B*, III, and V) ;
  1. the arms stretched,
  2. the arms bent, and the elbows reaching over the shoulders,
  3. the arms bent, and the lower part of them resting on the bars.

c. On the same bar, from before the hands to behind them, and the reverse, on the right, and left bar, (Compare Exerc. *B*, VI) ;
    1. the arms stretched,
    2. the arms bent, and the elbows reaching over the shoulders,
    3. the arms bent, and the lower part of them resting on the bars.

d. from one bar, before the hands, to the other, behind the hands, and the reverse, right and left (Compare Exerc. *B*, VII) ;
    1. the arms stretched,
    2. the arms bent, and the elbows reaching over the shoulders,
    3. the arms bent, and the lower part of them resting on the bars.

II. The gymnick rests on his hands (see pl. II, fig. 3), at the end of the bars, and after a few swings, or vibrations, the legs being closed, and stretched, *swings over the bar, before the arms*, the hand opposite to the side where the descent is made, pushing off, so that he comes to stand on the outside of the bars. The movement is corresponding to the fourth vault from the side (see page 27, IV), and ninth vault from behind (see page 32, IX). In descending on the right side, the left hand, in descending on the left, the right hand should take hold of the bar. The descent in this, and all other exercises, must be light, and on the toes. This exercise may be performed,
    a. the arms being stretched,
        1. over the right,
        2. over the left bar ;
    b. the arms being bent, and the elbows reaching over the shoulders,
        1. over the right,
        2. over the left bar ;

c. the arms being bent, and the lower part of them resting on the bars,
    1. over the right,
    2. over the left bar.

III. The gymnick rests on his hands (see pl. II, fig. 3), in the middle of the bars, and after a few vibrations, the legs being closed, and stretched, *swings over the bar, behind the arms*, the hand, opposite to the side where the descent is made, pushing off, so that he comes to stand on the outside of the bars. The movement is corresponding to the fifth vault from the side (see page 27, V), and tenth vault from behind (see page 33, X). In descending, which is made in an arch, as high and far from the bars as possible, no taking hold of the bars is required, or even possible. This exercise may be performed,

  a. the arms being stretched,
    1. over the right,
    2. over the left bar;

  b. the arms being bent, and the elbows reaching over the shoulders,
    1. over the right,
    2. over the left bar;

  c. The arms being bent, and the lower part of them resting on the bars,
    1. over the right,
    2. over the left bar.

IV. *Changing the seat, from one bar over the other, before the hands* (see Exerc. B, I, *a*, page 88), *with alighting* (see Exerc. B, II, page 89). It may be performed,

  a. the arms being stretched, alighting
    1. over the right,
    2. over the left bar;

  b. the arms being bent, and the elbows reaching over the shoulders, alighting
    1. over the right,
    2. over the left bar;

c. the arms being bent, and the lower part of them resting on the bars, alighting
 1. over the right,
 2. over the left bar.

V. *Changing the seat, from one bar over the other, behind the hands* (see Exerc. B, I, b, page 88) *with alighting* (see Exerc. B, III, page 90). It may be performed,
 a. the arms being stretched, alighting
  1. over the right,
  2. over the left bar;
 b. the arms being bent, the elbows reaching over the shoulders, alighting
  1. over the right,
  2. over the left bar;
 c. the arms being bent, the lower part of them resting on the bars, alighting
  1. over the right,
  2. over the left bar.

VI. *Changing the seat, on the same bar, from before the hands, to behind them, and the reverse* (see Exerc. B, I, c, page 89) *with alighting* (see Exerc. B, II, or III, page 89, and 90);
 a. forwards, from before the hands to behind the hands (see Exerc. B, I, c, page 89), and alighting before the hands (see Exerc. B, II, page 89);
  1. the arms being stretched,
   on the right,
   on the left bar;
  2. the arms being bent, and the elbows reaching over the shoulders,
   on the right,
   on the left bar;
  3. the arms being bent, and the lower part of them resting on the bars,
   on the right,
   on the left bar;
 b. backwards, from behind the hands to before them

(see Exerc. *B*, I, *c*, page 89), and alighting behind the hands (see Exerc. *B*, III, page 90);

    1. the arms being stretched,
        on the right,
        on the left bar;

    2. the arms being bent, and the elbows reaching over the shoulders,
        on the right,
        on the left bar;

    3. the arms being bent, and the lower part of them resting on the bars,
        on the right,
        on the left bar.

VII. *Changing the seat from one bar, before the hands, to the other, behind the hands, and the reverse* (see Exerc. *B*, I, *d*, page 89) *with alighting* (see Exerc. *B*, II, or III, page 89, and 90);

    a. forwards, from one bar, before the hands, to the other behind the hands (see Exerc. *B*, I, *d*, page 89), and alighting, before the hands (see Exerc. *B*, II, page 89);

    1. the arms being stretched, the movement beginning, and terminating
        on the right,
        on the left bar;

    2. the arms being bent, and the elbows reaching over the shoulders, the movement beginning, and terminating
        on the right,
        on the left bar;

    3. the arms being bent, and the lower part of them resting on the bars, the movement beginning, and terminating
        on the right,
        on the left bar;

b. backwards, from one bar, behind the hands, to the other, before the hands (see Exerc. *B*, I, *d*, page 89),

and alighting behind the hands (see Exerc. *B*, III, page 90);
   1. the arms being stretched, the movement beginning, and terminating
      on the right,
      on the left bar;
   2. the arms being bent, and the elbows reaching over the shoulders, the movement beginning, and terminating
      on the right,
      on the left bar;
   3. the arms being bent, and the lower part of them resting on the bars, the movement beginning, and terminating
      on the right,
      on the left bar.

VIII. The gymnick rests on his arms (see pl. II, fig. 3), in the middle of the bars, and throws his legs, straight, and in a straddling position over one bar, from thence in the same way over the other, so that always one leg is between, and the other without the bars. This may be done
   a. behind the arms,
   b. before the arms.

IX. *Circle;* a semicircular line, described with one leg over one bar, forwards and backwards.
   a. The gymnick rests on his arms (see pl. II, fig. 3), raises one leg forwards, passes it over the bar, describing a semicircle (see preparatory Exerc. page 5, at the bottom), the hand being lifted, and closes his legs This is from within to without.
   b. The reverse of it, or the circle from without to within, is, when the gymnick raises one leg backwards, passes it over the bar, describing a semicircle, and closes his legs. Both kinds should be practised.
      1. at the end of the bars,
         with the right,

with the left leg;

2. in the middle of the bars,
with the right,
with the left leg.

X. *Swinging.* (Compare Vaulting, first vault from behind, page 29). The gymnick rests upon his hands, (see pl. II, fig. 3), and puts his lower limbs in a vibrating motion; in swinging forwards, the belly is drawn in and the hips bent, in swinging backwards, the back is drawn in. An upright, and unaffected carriage of the head, pressing down, and keeping back the shoulders, are principal points to be attended to. (see pl. II, fig. 7.).

There are various kinds of *swinging*, which may be compounded differently; we shall mention only the most important:

a. as described above, *the arms being stretched*;

b. *with bending the arms, forward*; the moment, when the body, swinging backwards, has passed between the arms, they begin to bend as low as can possibly be done without turning over; and stretch again, as soon as the legs begin to swing forwards, so that the arms are stretched just when the body passes between them;

c. *with bending the arms, backwards*; the moment when the body, swinging forwards, has passed between the arms, these begin to bend so low, that the elbows are higher than the shoulders, and stretch again, as soon as the legs begin to swing backwards, so that the arms are stretched just when the body passes between them;

d. *with bending the arms, forwards and backwards*, a combination of the two preceding kinds (*b*, and *c*). In order to perform this exercise, it is necessary to have the arms stretched, each time when the body is passing between them;

e. *with bending the arms in the middle of the swing, backwards*, a movement opposite to the swinging *b*, in which the arms are stretched in the middle of the circular line, described by the movement of the body. The arms bend, when the legs begin to swing backwards, so that the elbows are lower than the shoulders, when the body passes between the arms. At the time the legs have reached the highest point of the swing, that is to say, when they are about to swing forwards, the arms must be stretched;

f. with bending the arms in the middle of the swing, forwards, a movement opposite to the swinging *c*, in which the arms are stretched in the middle of the circular line, described by the movement of the body. The arms begin to bend, when the legs begin to swing forwards, so that the elbows are lower, than the shoulders, when the body passes between the arms. At the time, when the legs are about to swing backwards, the arms must be stretched;

g. with bending the arms in the middle of the swing, backwards and forwards, a combination of the two preceding kinds. Particular attention must be paid to having the arms stretched at the beginning, and end of each swing;

h. with straddling at the end, *or* beginning, or at the end, *and* beginning of the swing.

i. with kicking at the end, *or* beginning, or at the end, *and* beginning of the swing. After the body has passed between the arms, the legs are bent in the knees and hips, (the same position as in the preparatory exercise Crouching, page 3, V), and vehemently thrown out, when the swing has reached the highest point. It must be exercised gradually, and with caution, because the kicking gives a violent shake to the whole body, especially to the arms.

h. with straddling, and kicking, a combination of *h,* and *i.*

It is well to practise these different kinds of *swinging*, at first, at the end of the bars, then, after having obtained sufficient dexterity, in the middle.

XI. A combination of *lowering upon the elbows, and rising*, with *swinging*;

a. backwards. The gymnick rests on his arms, (see pl. II, fig. 3), at the end of the bars, with his back towards the bars, bends both his arms, so as to rest with the lower part of them on the bars (see Exerc. *A*, IV, *b*, page 86), in this position swings backwards, and at the same time stretches his arms, gliding, with his hands, along the bars, bends again, and so on. The longer the gliding motion, the better;

b. forwards. The gymnick, as in *a*, resting with the lower part of his arms on the bars, swings forwards, and, at the same time, stretches his arms, gliding, with his hands, along the bars, bends again, and so on. The longer the gliding motion, the better.

XII. A combination of *moving along upon the hands*, (see Exerc. *A*, VIII, page 87), with *swinging*;

a. forwards. The gymnick rests on his arms (see pl. II, fig. 3), swings forwards, and, at the same time, moves, with his hands, along the bars; he continues this movement, till he has reached the end. The fewer strides, the better;

b. backwards. The gymnick rests on his hands, the back towards the bars, swings backwards, and, at the same time, moves, with his hands, along the bars.

XIII. *Swinging off:*

a. backwards. The gymnick rests on his arms (see pl. II, fig. 3), at the end of the bars, swings backwards, and pushes himself, horizontally, off (compare Vaulting, first vault from behind, page 29). Any one must bound back, at least, as much as the length of his body with his arms stretched;

b. forwards. The gymnick rests on his arms, with his back towards the bars, swings forwards, and pushes himself off.

In both kinds the gymnick should come to stand firmly on his feet.

XIV. *Turning over:*

a. from a suspended position. The gymnick, standing with his face towards the bars, takes hold of the bars, at the end, from beneath; the legs are thrown over backwards; after having touched, or nearly touched, the ground, they return the same way.

b. from the rest; at the end of the bars, the face outwards. The gymnick swings several times, the last time, backwards, so high, as to turn over, and to come to stand before the bars, in the same direction as at the commencement. This exercise must, at first, always be performed with the assistance of two persons, who take hold of the arms. Compare Vaulting, Exercises with the head foremost, fifth vault, page 48.

Pushing through, a good exercise for the back, but does not belong to either of the two kinds of exercises described under *A* and *B*. The gymnick stands on the side of the bars, takes hold of one bar, grasping from above, beneath, or either side, throws his legs under the first bar upon the second, pushes his body upon it as far as the back, and rises. The difficulty is greater, if the bars are narrow.

IX. CLIMBING.

Climbing is to endeavor to reach an elevated object which cannot be attained by means of the feet alone, by the assistance of the hands and feet, or hands alone.

Instruments:

1. *Climbing-pole,* from two to four inches thick, and proportional length, from ten to thirty feet high. It is best it should be made of the heart of strong wood, and planed.

2. *Climbing-mast,* from six to twelve inches thick, at the lower end, planed, and having, on the top, a cross, well fastened, to rest on. The height from 20 to 60 feet.

3. *Climbing-rope*, from 1 1-4 inches to 1 1-2 thick, with a loop, 20, 30, or 40 feet long.

4. *Ladders:*

a. wooden ladder, very firm, with well fixed flat rundles, the upper part of which must be rounded, so as not to offer any sharp edge, at no greater distance from one another than one foot. It is put up at an angle of 60°;

b. rope-ladder, twenty feet long; it is well, to have it with three wooden rundles, one at each end, and in the middle, to spread it out; it must be made so as not to twist, and entangle when used; else it becomes almost unserviceable.

5. *Slant*, or *oblique poles*, and *masts:* that is, poles, and masts which are fastened to a beam at an angle from 45° to 70°.

The fixing the instruments for climbing, is various. Where there are tall, stout trees, the ropes, poles, and masts, may be fastened to the limbs, or to beams, laid between the limbs. Where there are no such trees, instruments must be erected, on which several can exercise at the same time. All such instruments consist of two, three, four, or more perpendicular masts, connected by beams, to which ropes, ladders, and poles are fixed.

The description of some, already proved useful by experience, here follows.

1. *Single mast* (see pl. VIII, fig. R). A stout mast, 40 feet high, is set into the ground, with two horizontal beams at the upper end, reaching forth, on one side, six feet, and joined by a round piece of wood to which the rope is fixed. A slant ladder, standing six feet below, against the mast, supports the ends of the two beams. The beams reach forth, on the other side, three feet, and are supported by props, fastened to the mast. These beams are, near to the mast, and at the end, joined by boards, eight inches broad; the middle space of 20 inches remains open for passing through. From this opening a ladder, almost perpendicu-

lar, reaches down, 15 feet, to another standing-place, or platform, which is, therefore, 25 feet above the ground. From thence a ladder, as described above, extends to the ground, in an angle of 60°, which must be supported, in the middle, by props. Two more props may go up from the ground to the height of 25 feet, both to keep the mast steady, and to serve as slant poles for climbing.

2. *Climbing-stand of two masts* (see pl. VIII, fig. S). Two masts are set into the earth, at a distance of 18 feet from one another. They are joined, 20 feet above the ground, by a very strong cross-beam, reaching over on both sides from four to five feet. To either arm of the beam, a rope is fastened. A rope-ladder is hung in the middle; two poles, three inches thick, are erected in the space between the rope-ladder and the masts. Two slant poles lean on one side, two climbing-ladders on the other, against the masts.

3. *Climbing-stand of four masts* (see pl. VIII, fig. T). A very stout mast is set into the ground. Thirty feet above the ground, four beams, 12 feet long each, extend in the form of a cross, which, at a distance of eight feet from the main-mast, are supported by climbing masts. A rope is fixed to the arm of each beam. A climbing-ladder is placed in one of the angles, formed by the beams. Four feet from the masts, poles may be fixed.

4. An instrument, which is not altogether necessary, but which ought not to be omitted in a completely furnished gymnasium, is the following (see pl. VIII, fig. V), for climbing by means of the arms alone, forming a quadrangle of nine feet square. In the corners, four strong posts are fixed in the ground, and, six feet above the ground, are connected by four cross-pieces. A quadrangular frame is erected upon these cross-pieces, inclining at an angle of 60°. The four corner-posts of this frame are, in the way of a ladder, connected, foot by foot, by rundles five of which, on each side, are enough. These rundles are flat, at the lower part, at the upper rounded, and thinner, in order to afford an easy grasp.

All climbing is of two kinds:

A. climbing, properly so called, *with hands and feet.* This is either

    a. climbing in a hanging position, where the body has a position perpendicular, or inclined backwards; or

    b. climbing in a riding position, where the body has a position inclined forwards, and can hold itself by means of the feet alone.

B. Climbing by means of the arms alone, which is always climbing in a hanging position.

A. CLIMBING, PROPERLY SO CALLED.

Directions for climbing.

If the instrument for climbing is thin (as rope, and pole), the hands must do the most, and, therefore, grasp very firmly (see pl. II, fig. 8, and 9); if it cannot be clasped by the hand (as the mast), the hands with the lower part of the arms must be pressed against it, and the chest must make the reaction from the other side (see pl. II, fig. 10). If the mast is thick, the climber lays hold with one hand of the other arm; if it is very thick, the fingers of both hands may be interlaced.

The legs are placed around the mast, or pole, so that one presses from before with the calf, and heel, the other from behind with the instep, shin, and knee (see pl II, fig. 9, and 10). If the mast is thick, and rough, knees, and thighs, one from each side, close, the shins are laid on backwards and the toes press from behind. If the mast is very thick and smooth, when the fingers are interlaced, it is best to stretch the legs forward, and twist the feet also (see pl. II, fig. 10).

The rope is commonly taken hold of, only, by pressing it between the heel of one foot, and the instep of the other (see pl. II, fig. 8). Another method is this: the rope passes down from the hands of the climber along one thigh, not far above the knee winds around the inner-side of this thigh, along the knee-hollow and calf, and then across the instep whence it hangs loose. If the climber only treads, moderately, with the other foot, upon the rope where it crosses the instep, he will, by means of the varied pressure, obtain a firm support. The whole depends almost entirely upon holding the leg, and foot so that the rope may retain its proper winding, after being quitted by the other foot.

In climbing the hands rise alternately, one taking hold above the other, not one after the other.

In climbing, especially on the rope, all depends on the hands taking hold as high as possible, and then the feet being drawn up, near to the hands.

In *climbing down*, or *descending* the rope, the hands are never to be allowed to slide, but must make single grasps, as in climbing up. On the mast, and pole, sliding down may be allowed, but still with some caution, on account of the friction.

Climbing :

I. *on the pole*, is always climbing in a hanging position, and the easiest kind ; considerable dexterity, therefore, is to be acquired in it (see pl. II, fig. 9) ;

II. *on the mast*, is always climbing in a hanging situation, and the most difficult kind ; it affects the whole body very much, if the mast is high, and thick (see pl. II, fig. 10) ;

III. *on the slant pole*, is

    a. on the upper-side, climbing in a riding situation,

    b. on the under-side, climbing in a hanging position ;

the former of which, is the same movement as, in the common kind, described above ; the latter is various, depending chiefly on the different inclination, and size, of the pole.

IV. *on the rope ;* is always climbing in a hanging position :

    a. on the taught rope,

    b. on the loose rope,

    c. on the obliquely taught rope.

The most common, and convenient method of climbing on such a rope is,

    to throw the legs, after having taken hold with the hands, from both sides across the rope (compare the

Exercises on the single bar, Exerc. *A*, page 60), place, alternately, one hand beyond the other, and follow with the legs either in a sliding way,

or throwing, alternately, one leg over the rope, whilst the other is hanging down,

or sliding along only with one leg, whilst the other is hanging down,

or placing the sole of one foot flat upon the rope, and the other leg across the instep of that foot, and sliding thus along.

The most difficult climbing on a rope is with two feet, and one hand. Almost as difficult is, climbing in a reversed position; feet up, head below.

V. *on the ladder;*

a. on the rope-ladder, is the most difficult climbing of this kind, on account of the ladder being not fastened at the lower end, and the rundles being flexible. Before the pupil learns to support himself by his feet, he is obliged to bear almost his whole weight on his arms alone, the body at every step inclining backwards;

b. on the under side of the wooden ladder;

c. on the upper side, or front part of the wooden ladder. This cannot, properly, be styled climbing, but ascending, since the whole weight of the body is borne by the feet. Yet we may include it here; for the reason of its being a very good preparatory exercise for all kinds of climbing, on account of its accustoming the climber to be in an elevated place without becoming dizzy. The pupil should take hold of the sides of the ladder, not of the rundles.

1. Ascending, and descending with both hands. Descending with the back, or the face towards the ladder.

2. Ascending, and descending with one hand. After some time, it may be practised to carry something in the other.

3. Ascending, and descending without using the hands.

B. CLIMBING BY MEANS OF THE ARMS ALONE.

Since, in this exercise, the body is raised by means of the hands alone, the legs, and the rest of the body must be kept as quiet as possible.

The exercise *A*, VI, (page 64), on the single bar, is the best preparatory exercise.

All *climbing by means of the arms alone*, is either:

I. with a grasp, where the plane of the hand is perpendicular, on perpendicular, or slant ropes; or

II. with a grasp, where the plane of the hand is horizontal, on horizontal instruments for climbing.

I. The climbing with a grasp, where the plane of the hand is perpendicular, is always done, one hand grasping above, not after the other; the elbows must be as close to the body as possible. The body can be

    a. perfectly straight,
    b. bent in the knees,
    c. bent in the knees, and hips,
    d. bent in the hips.

The legs can be kept

    a. closed on one side,
    b. straddling on both sides of the pole, or rope.

This kind of climbing is practised:

    a. on the rope, both perpendicular, and slant,
    b. on the pole, and slant pole, provided that they can be grasped;
    c. on the two main-ropes of the rope ladder.

II. The climbing with a grasp, where the plane of the hand is horizontal, is done almost exclusively on the wooden ladder, or the instrument, described page 99, 4. It being extremely difficult on the rope-ladder, on account of the flexibility of the rundles. It ought to be practised, one hand grasping beyond the other; this being, however, very difficult, it may be allowed to grasp with one hand after the other, provided it is not always done with the same hand, but with both hands alternately.

Climbing, where both hands at a time advance from one rundle to the other, is to be done only near to the ground, because grasping amiss is not uncommon.

Climbing on the instrument, described above, page 99, 4, is practised in the same way as on the ladder. The gymnick ascends on one side, and descends in the next, and so on, as long as his strength allows, without touching the ground. This instrument has this advantage over the ladder, that several can climb, at a time, and vie with each other in climbing.

For *climbing in emulation*, in general, at least two equally thick, and high poles (as on the instrument described page 99, 2), ropes (as on the instrument described page 99, 2, and 3), or masts are requisite.

Passing by one another in climbing may be done:
    a. in climbing up, and
    b. in climbing down, or descending.

It is commonly a mixture of the first (*A*), and second (*B*) kind of climbing.

X. THROWING.

There are *six* kinds of throwing:
  A. Shooting:
    1. with fire-arms,
    2. with the cross-bow,
    3. with the bow,
    4. with the dart.

B. Throwing heavy bodies, done by a simple swinging, forwards and backwards, of the arm stretched.

C. Throwing, or throwing heavy bodies by stretching the arm after bending.

D. Throwing an iron bar.

E. Slinging, or throwing light bodies by various kinds of swinging, by means either of the hands alone, or of particular instruments.

F. *Ricocheter.*
G. *Throwing ducks, and drakes.*

Throwing is one of the most important exercises, both for strengthening the arms, and sharpening the eye-sight; it requires, however, great precaution, much space, and possibility of calculating the movement of the body thrown. Only the kinds *A,* 4, *B, C,* and *D,* can be practised in the gymnasium, and ought by no means to be omitted, though they are not suited for children under eleven years.

A. SHOOTING.

1. *With fire-arms,* especially the rifle, is an excellent exercise for youths. It would be very desirable to have a particular shooting-place connected with every gymnasium, where youths could receive instruction at particular hours, since the usual time for gymnastick exercises, would be too much disturbed by this exercise. It cannot be the object to form good riflemen, for this requires long practice; but every one ought to have a familiar acquaintance with fire-arms, and know how to use them.

Instruments:

a. The rifle. It cannot be our object, to give a description of this ingenious piece of mechanism, but every one, using a rifle, ought to be acquainted with its construction, in order to use it advantageously, especially to know, in what particular way, it carries the shot.

b. The aim:

1. a board, round, two feet in diameter, the centre of which, five inches in diameter, is black, and surrounded by twelve parallel circles, at equal distance from one another. It is fixed to a post, so that its lower circumference is three feet from the ground;

2. a box, quadrilateral, each side four feet square, supported by three or four posts, so that the different sides can easily be turned towards the shooter, three feet from the ground. The first side is divided by a perpen-

dicular mark, three inches broad; the second has a perpendicular cross, both lines of which are three inches broad; the third side has a number of quadrangles, one contained in the other, so that their sides are parallel, at a distance of three inches from one another; the fourth has a number of circles, one contained in the other, distant three inches from one another. The inner space of the box is filled with sand, and thus preserves the balls which reach the aim;

3. a board, which can be put in motion, six feet high, the upper half of which is divided into three equal parts, one foot three inches broad, which breadth is divided into three spaces, that in the centre nine inches broad.

c. The *post*, to lean against with the rifle, with holes bored through, beginning four feet from the ground, distant two inches from one another, in which a wooden peg fits.

The place, behind the aim, is surrounded by a mound of turf, 20 feet long, 12 feet high.

Charging:

Some tow is put in the pan, and the latter shut. The rifle is put to the ground, so that it is held by the knees, the barrel turned towards the body, the gunstick outwards, and the muzzle away from the gymnick. The powder, which should be measured very exactly (the seventh part of the weight of the ball), is poured into the barrel, upon the powder; the ball, enveloped in the patch, consisting of a piece of cotton so large as to cover two thirds of the ball, and greased on the outside, is pushed down with the gunstick, so that it sits closely upon the powder. To ascertain whether there is no empty space left between the powder and ball, the gunstick is thrown in, the rifle being lifted, and as soon as it rebounds, the ball sits fast. The rifle is taken up, the butt-end placed under the right arm, the pan opened, and filled with powder, care being taken that the communication with the barrel through the touch-hole is kept up by some grains of powder. After the shot, the cock, flint, and pan are to be cleaned with a piece of cloth, the touch-hole with a feather. There is no need of cleaning the barrel each time, if the charge is immediately renewed.

Posture:

The heels stand on the same line, about one foot distant from each other, the toes outwards; the upper part of the body, and the head erect. The left hand takes hold of the rifle, close to the lowest loop, the thumb on the left side, and stretched, the first two fingers on the right side, and laid down. The right hand grasps with the last three fingers the back-part of the triggerguard, the first finger rests on the fore-part of it, the thumb is laid over the neck of the stock. Thus the rifle is raised so high, that the cheek-piece comes to rest on the right cheek, and the breech on the right shoulder, preserving the horizontal direction of the aim, without bending the head.

Aiming:

Aiming is to bring the after-sight, and the fore-sight in one straight line, directed upon the object to be shot at. It depends upon the peculiarity of the rifle, and the distance of the object, whether the whole fore-sight, or half of it, or only the head, is to be seen in the after-sight.

Preparatory Exercises:

I. The gymnick endeavors to bring the ball always in the same perpendicular line, avoiding its deviating to the right, or left side. The first side of the box, described under *b*, 2 (page 105), serves as an aim for this exercise.

II. The gymnick endeavors to bring the ball always in the same horizontal line, avoiding its deviating upwards, or downwards. The second side of the bar, described under *b*, 2 (page 105), serves as an aim.

III. A combination of the two preceeding exercises (I, and II). The second, and third sides of the bar, described under *b*, 2 (page 105), serve as aims for this exercise.

All these exercises are performed:

a. with resting on, and leaning against the post, described under *c* (page 106), so that the barrel rests on, and the highest loop presses lightly against, the peg of the post;

b. with resting on the peg of the post. In order to prevent leaning against the peg, the latter may be covered with a roller, which turns at the least pressure from the side;

c. with resting on the right side of the post, without using the peg.

Exercises:

I. The gymnick endeavors to bring the ball into the centre of the round board, described under *b*, 1 (page 105); or into the centre of the third side of the bar, described under *b*, 2 (page 105);

a. with resting on, and leaning against, the peg of the post;

b. with resting on the peg of the post;

c. with resting on the post.

II. The preparatory exercise I (page 107), without resting, or leaning on; at arm's length.

III. The preparatory exercise II (page 107), without resting, or leaning on; at arm's length.

IV. The preparatory exercise III (page 107), without leaning, or resting on; at arm's length.

V. The first exercise, without leaning, or resting on; at arm's length.

VI. The gymnick endeavors to bring the ball into the upper part of the moveable board, described under *b*, 3 (page 106);

a. with resting on, and leaning against, the peg of the post;

b. with resting on the peg of the post;

c. with resting on the post;

d. without leaning, or resting on; at arm's length.

VII. The gymnick, lying on the ground, supported by his elbows, and resting his rifle upon his hat, endeavors to bring his ball into the different aims described above.

Precautions:

a. The gymnick should avoid moving about, after the rifle has been charged, hold the muzzle towards the ground, never towards a person;

b. should not set the hair-trigger, before he has taken his aim;

c. should not carry his rifle charged without covering the flint with a leathern cap.

B. *With the cross-bow.* This, if good, can almost supply the place of fire-arms; but then it is expensive, and requires likewise much precaution; fire-arms therefore are to be preferred. Shooting with the cross-bow, however, is a very pleasant exercise, and useful for boys.

C. *With the bow.* This kind of shooting, is a very useful exercise, making a steady arm, and a sharp eye; it is equally useful for persons of every age, and, therefore, much to be commended out of the gymnasium.

Instruments:

a. The bow. The best wood for a bow is the greater maple, soft maple, falsely called Sycamore (acer pseudoplataneis), or the Norway maple (acer platanoides), or the common or lesser maple (acer campestre), or the common holly (ilex aquifolia), and before all the common yew (taxus baccata). It is best to cut the wood, destined for a bow, in the winter, and to choose a stick which is of nearly equal thickness at both ends, and without knots, at least on that part which is to be the outside. The middle, for taking hold of the bow, is left unwrought, unless it be too thick, in which case on the inside some wood is cut off, without altering the round shape. Both horns, or ends, are wrought flat, and decreasing towards the ends. Care must be taken that no part is weaker than the rest. Then it is fixed in a position somewhat curved, and left to dry. The ends may easily be turned outwards a little, if the wood, when yet green, is heated over fire, and forced into that form. When the wood is dried, the string is fixed to it. The length of the bow is from three to six feet. If it is considerably curved, it ought not to be very long, on account of its requiring too long arrows. A good bow must be elastic and flexible, but not stiff. The string is made of hemp or catgut.

b. The arrow; is best of wood which splits straight, planed round and smooth; it must be perfectly straight. The point is covered with horn, bone, tin, or iron; the other end has a cleft, to lay it on the string. The arrow, when feathered, carries much farther. This is done in the following manner. The feathers from the tail of a bird, because they are straight, are taken, best of a bird of prey; the beard is drawn from the quill, and fixed, in stripes of three inches long, to the lower end of the arrow, either along the axis on two sides, or in a spiral line; in the former case the arrow is carried straight, in the latter, it turns around its axis. The feathers ought not to be longer than 1-4 or 1-3 of an inch.

Holding the bow:

The gymnick takes hold of the bow, in the middle, the arm being stretched, more or less approaching a perpendicular direction, never in a horizontal. The arrow is put on the string at the cleft end, the other rests on the thumb, or between the first two fingers of the left hand. The thumb and the first finger of the right hand take hold of the lower end, and draw it, quick and strongly, back with the string, which sends the arrow off, as soon as the fingers loosen their grasp.

Aiming is not so much that of the cross-bow or rifle, as a quick, and intuitive as it were computation of the distance, elastic power of the bow, and weight of the arrow, a kind of tact obtained by long practice.

The perpendicular shot is to be avoided; it carries the arrow to a great height, and this can, even when blunt, enter the skull.

B. *With the dart, or darting.*

Instruments:

a. The dart (see pl. VII, fig. C) is a perfectly straight shaft. The point is provided with an iron plate four inches long, which terminates hemispherically or conically (see pl. VII. fig. C, *a*). The other end is furnished with an iron ring, two inches long (see pl. VII, fig. C, *b*), which must have so much counterpoise, as to bring the point of gravity but two or three inches from the middle towards the point.

For boys under twelve years, the dart should be six feet long, and one inch, or, at the most, 1 1-4 inches thick; for larger and older persons, in proportion to their strength, seven or eight feet long, and 1 1-4 or 1-2 inches thick. No darts of another size should be used. Dry wood should be employed for darts, if possible ash; but if this cannot be obtained, pine will answer.

b. The stake as aim (see pl. VII, fig. B). A wooden block, from 12 to 16 inches high, similar in shape to a head (see pl. VII, fig. B, *a*), is fastened, by a cramp-iron, to a post, four feet or four feet and 1-2 high, from five to six inches thick (see pl. VII, fig. B, *b*). The cramp-iron is fixed by two strong iron rings, both to the head and the post, so that the head, if hit, turns over, but remains hanging on the post.

The ground, intended for this exercise (see pl. VII, fig. 13), must be at least 30 feet wide, on account of the darts frequently rebounding far. At the end of this place a mound, three or four feet high, is thrown up, 20 feet from which, at least, the stake is placed. A fence of planks is still better, because the darts, sometimes, when thrown violently and straight, slip over the mound. From 40 to 50 feet are necessary for a shot without a run, so that the whole ground must be 70 feet long.

Position of the thrower:

Feet are placed separate; the foot on the same side with the arm throwing, behind and across; the other foot on the same side with the arm resting, before, and turned a little outwards.

The arm resting, in a sharp angle, the hand closed, the nails towards the face.

The arm throwing, in a sharp angle, the dart held with the

fist in a balancing position, near to the face (see pl. VI, fig. 1). Both feet immoveable on the ground.

Preparatory exercises.

I. Finding the point of gravity of the dart.

II. Holding, and carrying the dart in a balancing position, in standing, and running.

III. Moving the dart, by a sudden start, backwards, in a perpendicular position.

IV. Moving the dart, by a sudden start, forwards, in a perpendicular position, without loosening the fingers.

V. Combining the two movements III, and IV, and practising them repeatedly, as quickly and strenuously as possible.

VI. Throwing, at first short, then longer, all the fingers quitting the dart at a time.

Exercises.

A throw is either in a *straight,* curved, or *declining* line.

1. The *throw in a straight line,* or the level shot, is made in conformity to the manner of holding the dart, described above (see page 111 ; pl. VI, fig. 1), and the preparatory exercises (see page 112), horizontal, as much so as the law of gravity allows. Some dexterity must be obtained in this throw, before the pupil passes to the next.

II. The *throw in a curved line* requires less strength, but more practice and dexterity. The dart is taken hold of so that it has some overweight towards the point (see pl. VI, fig. 2). The skill consists in giving the dart, at the moment of throwing, such a push that, having reached the proper height, it sinks with the point foremost. The angle in which the dart descends, must be under 45°, else it turns over, and has too little effect.

There are two principal methods of holding the dart.

a. The arm is, at the commencement of the throw, almost entirely stretched, and turned so that the opening of the fingers is above ; the breast is turned a little towards the dart. This is the most common mode.

b. The arm is, at the commencement of the throw, less stretched, and not turned at all; neither is the breast turned, but the upper part of the body inclines much backwards. This mode of throwing affects the body very much.

The throw in a curved line reaches farther, than that in a straight. It should be practised with regard first to height alone, and then to height and distance together.

III. The *throw in a declining line* can be either
in a straight or
curved line.

All three kinds of throws can be performed:
  a. as to the posture,
    1. from the spot, or standing,
    2. with a run;
  b. as to the arms,
    1. with the right arm,
    2. with the left arm, which must be practised just as well as with the right, in all kinds of throwing.

Thus twelve variations arise.

The mark can be considered hit, only when the point touches.

If the dart, in throwing, instead of pursuing its proper line, straight or curved, wavers and shakes, and if it touches with the shaft instead of the point, it is to be considered a false throw.

B. THROWING BY MEANS OF SWINGING THE ARM STRETCHED FORWARDS AND BACKWARDS.

This is a mode of throwing where the bodies to be thrown are placed in the hand as balls in the play at nine pins. Since throwing at a mark is to be practised in the gymnasium, cannon-balls, from one to three pounds weight, are only to be used. Balls of one pound and a half or two pounds, are the most convenient for this kind of throwing.

The place, intended for this exercise (see pl. VII, fig. 14), must be from 16 to 20 feet wide, and have, besides, free space on both sides so that the line of throwing is, on either side, distant 30 feet from all places for other exercises; the whole width, therefore, is 60 feet. The length is 100 feet.

The mark (see pl. VII, fig. 14, *a*), consists of a frame, eight or nine feet high, four feet wide, of wood four or five inches broad. In the centre a bag entirely filled with sand, or stuffed, is hung up, which, being hit, gives way. Six or eight feet behind the mark, a mound, covered with strong planks, with two wings, the higher the better (see pl. VII, fig. 14, *b*), is erected, so that the balls roll back. Behind this mound a space of 20 feet, surrounded with a low mound, (see pl. VII, fig. 14, *c*), must be left unoccupied, on account of the balls, which may, perhaps, be thrown over the mound. Thus the whole place has a breadth of 60, and a length of 130 feet.

Position:

The foot on the side of the arm throwing stands back and across, the other forwards and straight out. The arm throwing is held down on the thigh of the same side; the wrist is considerably bent. The other arm rests with the hand upon the other thigh (see pl. VI, fig. 3).

Method of throwing:

The hand throwing takes hold of the ball, the arm, after swinging several times forwards and backwards, the body not inclining forwards or backwards, throws; the ball must leave the hand and fingers at the same time. It is thrown right and left, by turns. The thrower stands in the middle of the place; the lookers on, or the partakers of the same exercise, stand on the side opposite to the arm throwing, lest they should be injured.

A kind of throwing, similar to this, but scarcely to be practised in a gymnasium, on account of the large space required, is the throwing of a wooden, stony, or iron *quoit* (or rather *discus*), which must revolve around its own axis whilst passing through the air.

C. THROWING BY STRETCHING THE ARM WHICH WAS BEFORE BENT.

Since this kind of throwing can never be used to hit a mark with certainty, and at a considerable distance, it serves chiefly to strengthen the arm, and is, therefore, practised in throwing heavy weights straight forwards, or downwards.

The place, destined for this exercise (see pl. VII, fig. 15), is from 20 to 30 feet wide, and 40 feet long. The standing-place, from six to eight feet broad, must be bounded by a tree, sunk horizontally half into the ground (see pl. VII, fig. 15, *a*) upon which, in throwing, the fore-foot is placed. The end of the place is limited by a low mound (see pl. VII, fig. 15, *b*) to prevent the balls rolling too far. It is well to have a ditch before the standing-place over which the balls are thrown.

Instrument :

Cannon-balls from 6 to 24 pounds, are the best implements for this kind of throwing, because they are easily held, and their weight is known.

Mode of throwing :

Carriage and position is the same as in the preceding exercise *B*, (see page 114). But the arm throwing is bent in a sharp angle, with the hand bent up, to the same height with the face. The ball is placed in the open hand and, after a few movements forwards and backwards of the body and arm, thrown off (see pl. VI, fig. 4).

The following exercise does not strictly belong to the class : throwing, but since it is the only exercise in pushing which can be practised in a gymnasium, we mention it :

A heavy beam which turns upon a stand about four feet high, in a balancing position, around a strong nail or peg, is put in motion by pushing. The force of the push is calculated by the number of revolutions of the beam, which may easily be counted by a simple contrivance.

D. THROWING AN IRON BAR.

Instrument:

An *iron bar*, about three feet long, and of different thickness, according to the strength of the person using it.

Posture:

The gymnick stands with his feet in one line, outwards, one foot about two feet from the other; the body erect, the right arm raised forwards in a horizontal line.

Exercise:

The right arm, the hand taking hold of the bar on its point of gravity, so that it easily preserves the perpendicular position into which it is brought at the beginning, swings twice or three times, without bending the elbows, from before the breast backwards, the upper part of the body turning to the right, as far as the joints of the shoulder will allow; the last time, in coming forwards, the hand loosens its grasp, and the bar is carried to some distance. The first object must be the bar preserving its perpendicular position during the whole movement so that it touches the earth with the lower end first; the second, to carry the bar as far as possible, opposite the front of the gymnick. The same is to be practised with the left arm.

E. SLINGING.

Throwing light bodies which are put in motion by means of the hands alone, or of particular instruments, by various kinds of swinging.

I. *Slinging by means of the hands alone*, or *common throwing*. The modes of throwing are very various; the most common are:

    a. the arm swings backwards and high;

    b. the arm swings backwards and low;

    c. the hand rests, at the beginning, with the wrist against the back.

This kind of throwing is practised with small stones, balls, and similar light bodies, not exceeding in weight half a pound, *from the spot or with a run*, in the following ways:

with a long throw,
with a high throw,
at an aim.

II. *Slinging by means of particular instruments,* as sling, stick, strap, string, etc.

No kind of slinging, as has been already mentioned, can be practised in the gymnasium.

F. RICOCHETER.

Throwing with a bounce upon the solid ground, cannot be practised in the gymnasium, because the direction cannot, with any degree of certainty, be calculated.

G. THROWING DUCKS AND DRAKES.

Throwing with a pebble, slate, or sherd upon the surface of water, so that the piece thrown, rebounding several times, glides along.

XI. DRAWING.

Instruments:

1. *A rope,* at least 20 feet long, and one inch thick, with loops on both ends. If thirty draw on each side, the rope must be 60 feet.

2. An instrument for drawing, (see pl. VII, fig O), consisting of two girths, from two to three feet long, and two or three inches broad, the ends of which are connected by two ropes, each 10 feet long.

3. *Staves* of birch, two or three feet long, and one fourth or half inch thick.

The *place,* intended for this exercise, must be level, and of a length proportional to the length of the ropes.

A. DRAWING WITH THE HANDS.

I. *With the hands alone;*

a. the hands take hold of one another, singly: the right of the right, the left of the left;

b. hooking:

1. singly, the right hand with the right, the left with the left;

2. doubly, the right hand hooking with the left, and the left with the right;
    with four fingers;
    with one finger.

II. *By means of instruments:*

a. On the rope, a contest in drawing; the hands take hold of the rope, the thumb turned against the adversary, and the steps retreat. The number on each side can be equal or odd. If there are many on each side, it is best to draw by jerks. A great assistance in doing this is, to number aloud. The contest in drawing can, therefore, be a contest
    of two,
    of three,
    of many.

Another mode of taking hold of the rope, if two persons are to draw, is to pass the rope over the shoulder of the arm which is not drawing, the hand of which takes hold of the end, across the back and below the arm drawing the hand of which, too, takes hold.

b. On the rope passing over a roller. The roller is fixed to a stand, particularly erected for this purpose, or a tree, about nine or ten feet from the ground. Two gymnicks take hold, one on each end, of the rope, and each endeavors to draw the other towards the roller, or even to raise him from the ground.

c. On the staff; a contest of two: one takes hold of the staff near to the ends, the other near to the middle.

Raising a person, lying on the ground, may be done in several ways, described above. The best method is: two sit down upon the earth, pressing with their soles against each other, and, taking hold of the staff, in the way described *A*, II, *b*, endeavor to raise one another.

B. DRAWING WITH THE NECK.

a. Standing; the instrument described under 2, (page 117), is stretched out; each one places a girth around his neck, facing his adversary, and endeavors to draw him away. Turning to either side, is not allowed, but the parties remain face to face. The hands are not to take hold of the ropes, but should be laid on the hips, the thumbs turned backwards, (see page 2).

b. Resting on hands and feet. The same instrument is stretched out. Each one steps with one foot over both ropes, back against back, places the girth around his neck, so that the ropes pass through between the legs, stoops down so as to rest on the hands, and endeavors to draw his adversary along, the back being stretched, and the head raised. This exercise is not dangerous, although it has that appearance to those who have not tried it.

All exercises in drawing have the advantage of not requiring preparatory exercises, so that even those, not yet practised, can immediately join them.

XII. PUSHING.

There are *two* kinds of *pushing*:

A. Pushing of an adversary, where force is employed against force;

 a. hand taking hold of hand,
  the right of the right,
  the left of the left;

the arms are perfectly stretched; the object is to compel the adversary to yield, or bend his arm.

 b. the hands placed upon each other's shoulders;

  1. the hands are placed before the pushing begins, either both on the inside of the other's arms, or on the outside, or one on the inside, the other on the outside;

  2. both endeavor to gain the best hold, (this is on the inside of the other's arms, because this is the shortest line from shoulder to shoulder).

This pushing is performed :

1. on both feet, with hold described under *b*, 1 and 2;

2. on one foot; either the stronger on one foot, or both.

B. Pushing on a particular instrument, where the weight alone of the object is to be overcome.

A waggon, with four wheels, on a solid smooth ground, loaded, according to the strength of the gymnick, with stones or cannon-balls, the weight of which is ascertained.

XIII. LIFTING.

All kinds of lifting heavy burdens, especially with legs separate, which affects the belly very much, are not suitable for the gymnasium. Lifting with arms perpendicularly stretched, which is very strengthening for the arms, belongs here.

I. *Lifting an instrument to measure the strength of the arms,* (dynameometron). There may be various kinds of such instruments; we shall describe only two :

a. *A staff,* (see pl. VII, fig. P), squared, four or five feet long, one inch thick, with notches, distant from one another one inch, and a handle, six inches long. Weights from one to two pounds, provided with rings, are hung on the notches.

b. A box, 15 inches 5-12 square, three inches high; the borders are 2-3 of an inch thick; the interior space is divided into 144 squares, one inch square each; the partitions are 1-4 of an inch thick, and need not reach to the bottom. The four squares in the centre are taken off to admit a handle, which is there firmly fixed in the bottom, and reaches eight inches over. Square pieces of iron, of a weight which can be multiplied without great fractions, are made to suit those squares. The weight of the box empty must be ascertained.

The former instrument a, is taken hold of so that the opening between the thumb and first finger is upwards, the fingers inwards. Arm and staff form a straight line. The staff, with a weight, according to the strength of the lifter, is slowly raised to a horizontal position, and lowered again. To lift a weight of two pounds at a distance of 50 inches from the hand, requires a considerable degree of strength. It increases the difficulty of the exercise, to keep the staff still for some time, when it has reached the horizontal line. It is practised:
  1. with one staff,
  2. with one staff in each hand.

The second instrument is filled with iron pieces, according to the strength of the pupil, equally on all sides, the squares near the centre first.

This exercise too, should be practised with both arms at a time. This is the best means to prevent any inclining or turning of the body, all of which should be carefully avoided.

II. *Lifting a balance-beam.* A heavy beam is placed, in equilibrium, upon a stand two or three feet high, on one side with a ring. This is taken hold of with the hand, the arm being stretched, and held, whilst the beam is removed from its point of gravity, or loaded with weights.

III. *Holding of sand-bags,* or rather *weights,* which are suspended on the stretched arms.

XIV. CARRYING.

Carrying must not be commenced till after some practice in other exercises. At the commencement the burden must be very inconsiderable, and increase very gradually with the increase of strength. To gain some facility in carrying, time, patience, habit, constant practice, and perseverance are requisite. The chief excellence consists in the ability to continue for a long time; and to have strength for other movements, at the same time.

A. CARRYING INANIMATE BODIES.

I. *Carrying with the hands:*
   a. With arms stretched out horizontally, holding sandbags.
   b. With arms kept down, holding guns, or heavy poles.

II. *Carrying on the shoulders:*
   a. guns, or heavy poles;
   b. a knapsack, with two straps, suspended on both shoulders, and of a weight not to prevent the performing of other exercises, hands and arms being free. However useful this exercise is, especially for journeys on foot, it becomes injurious to the chest, if heavy burdens are carried, and the exercise too long continued (see Walking, page 8).

B. CARRYING A MAN.

Only larger and stronger persons should carry smaller and lighter ones.

I. *On the back,* the thighs of the person borne resting on the hips of the person carrying.

II. *On the shoulders,* the thighs of the person borne resting on the shoulders of the person carrying.

III. *On the hands.* Two persons standing opposite take hold with their right hand of their own left wrist, and with their left hand of the other's right wrist, or vice versa;
   a. carrying a person sitting, by two;
   b. carrying a person lying, requires a line of couples. In this position the following exercise may be practised. All stretch their arms, at a time, and thus fling the person lying on their hands, into the air. At every fling the person carried advances one couple. Those under his head stretch their arms with most force.

XV. EXERCISES WITH DUMB-BELLS.

Instrument:

A pair of dumb-bells; they are too well known to require a particular description. We shall confine ourselves to one remark. The common kind of dumb-bells has a straight handle; it is better, to have the handle curved.

It is of great importance after the preparatory exercises have been sufficiently practised, to make use of very light dumb-bells, and to exchange them only after an apparent increase of strength, for those of greater weight. If this is not observed, the muscles will be exerted too much, and weakness, instead of increase of strength, be the consequence of this exercise.

PREPARATORY EXERCISES.

Posture:

Feet and knees close together, the whole body erect, breast outwards, shoulders drawn back; arms hanging down by the sides, the fingers being clenched, the thumb pressed upon them.

I. The right arm is thrown forwards the nails upwards, and backwards the knuckles upwards. The same is to be done with the left arm.

II. Both arms thrown forwards, at a time, the nails upwards.

III. The upper part of the arms are raised to a horizontal line, the elbows bent so that the hands approach the shoulders; the right hand is thrown out, so as to extend the arm at right angles to the side of the body, and bent again. The same is to be done with the left hand.

IV. Both hands are thrown out together.

V. The elbows, close to the body, are bent, so that the hands are as high as the arm-pits; the right hand is thrown forward, so that the whole arm forms a horizontal line, and bent again. The same is to be done with the left hand.

VI. Both hands are thrown forwards together, and bent again.

VII. The right arm is raised, so that the elbow is opposite the middle of the chest, and the hand touches the left shoulder; it is then thrown sideways, as if giving a broadsword-cut. The same is to be done with the left arm.

VIII. The arms, close to the body, are bent, the right arm is thrust up in a perpendicular direction, and bent again. The same is to be done with the left arm.

IX. Both arms are thrust up together, and bent again.

X. The upper part of the arms is raised sideways, the elbows bent, so that the hands come below the arm-pits; the right arm is thrust down in a perpendicular direction, and bent again. The same is to be done with the left arm.

XI. Both arms are thrust down together, and bent again.

XII. Both arms are thrust up, and bent again; then thrust down, and bent again.

XIII. The arms are stretched forwards, so that the palms touch, and swung backwards, in a horizontal plane, so that the knuckles touch, and again forwards.

XIV. The arms are stretched forward, so that the backs of the hands touch, and swung backwards, so that the palms touch.

XV. The arms are stretched downwards, the palms of the hands against the thighs, and raised, in a perpendicular plane, so that the knuckles touch above the head.

XVI. The right arm is raised forwards, and without bending, passed over backwards, as much as possible in a perpendicular plane, so that it describes a circle, the centre of which is the shoulder of the gymnick. The same is to be done with the left arm.

XVII. Both arms are raised together, so that they describe two parallel circles.

EXERCISES.

Most of the *preparatory exercises* described, may be performed with dumb-bells. Each hand takes hold of the handles of the dumb-bell. As to the movements themselves, they remain unaltered as they have been described. The following of the preparatory exercises are those which may be performed with dumb-bells: I, II, III, IV, V, VI, VII, VIII, IX, X, XI, XIII, XV, XVI, XVII.

XVI. WRESTLING.

The *place*, destined for this exercise, must be so large as to admit from four to six pairs, without disturbing each other. If several are to wrestle, the place must be from 60 to 100 feet long, and from 40 to 50 wide. The ground should be soft, and carefully cleared from all stones, roots, chips, and such things.

Position (see pl. VI, fig. 5):

One foot forwards towards the antagonist, the knee bent;
the other foot behind and across;
the elbows close to the body;
the fists clenched, before the body, close together;
upper part of the body inclining forwards.

Standing thus, the wrestler offers the greatest resistance for him who endeavors to lift him from the ground, or to push him from his place. The wrestler must never be in a high, erect posture, but rather low against his antagonist.

Grasp:

There are two kinds of grasp, or hold: the *entire*, and the *half grasp*.

The *entire grasp* is, seizing the antagonist around his waist, with both arms under his (see pl. VI, fig. 6);

the *half grasp* is, when one arm is over, the other under, that of the antagonist (see pl. VI, fig. 7).

In grasping around, the fingers should never be interlaced, because interlacing prevents the free use of the hands; but one hand can take hold of the wrist of the other, which, being closed, may serve to press against the back of the adversary, and to bend him down.

FIRST SECTION.

PREPARATORY EXERCISES.

I. Endeavoring to obtain the entire grasp.
II. Lifting the adversary from the ground.
III. Bending the back of the adversary.
IV. Laying down, right or left.

These three exercises, II, III, and IV, are to be practised with the entire, and half grasp; and the adversary either remaining quiet, or defending himself.

V. Holding down on the ground; particularly useful, when a stronger is kept down by a weaker one:

   a. extending the arms of the adversary lying on his back, and encompassing with the legs those of the adversary (see pl. VI, fig 8);

   b. lying down upon the adversary, chest upon chest, encompassing the upper part of the adversary's body with the half grasp, so that both form almost a right angle with their bodies. The same distance is kept, by removing, if the adversary should approach in order to take hold with his feet and to turn over (see pl. VI, fig. 9);

   c. two smaller ones, equal in strength to one larger; one takes hold of the adversary in the way described under *b*, the other encompasses his legs with his arms.

He that is lying on the ground, must endeavor

VI. to rise; if lying on his back, he must first seek to turn; then he can more easily rid himself from the hold of his adversary.

EXERCISES.

I. After these preparatory exercises, wrestling with the half grasp may be practised, to find out the weight and strength, without any regard to practice and dexterity in wrestling. The combatants stand opposite to each other, both holding the same arm up, and the other down, in a diagonal line, and so take equally hold of each other. Either both the right or both the left arms are upwards.

II. The wrestling with an equal grasp forms the transition to the wrestling without any previous agreement, or allowance on either side.

To represent and describe systematically wrestling, with attack and defence, grasp and counter-grasp, is not easy, since the number of grasps or holds is very great, and each counter-grasp influenced, or occasioned by the grasp of the antagonist, or other circumstances. Practice will very soon afford a familiar acquaintance with many different modes.

In a complete wrestle, not *throwing*, but *keeping down*, decides the contest, unless another criterion is before agreed upon.

It ought especially to be borne in mind, that every wrestle is a contest of strength, with the object of measuring and increasing strength and activity, not injuring the opponent. If this is well understood, no animosity will appear. According to this principle, it is not lawful:

to lay hold of the clothes merely, still less of the hair,
of single fingers;
to twist single limbs;
to push, or strike;
to bite, or scratch;
to grasp, passing with the arm between the thighs;
to kneel upon the chest, or any other part of the body of the adversary.

Wrestling may be exercised:
1. one against one,
2. one against two,
3. one against three,
4. many against many.

Those who are weak, stiff, clumsy, not yet experienced in gymnastic exercises, should not be admitted to wrestling.

No wrestle is to be performed without inspection.

No wrestle should be continued to the exhaustion of either of the combatants.

Whenever one of the wrestlers begins to become angry, the wrestle should be immediately stopped.

XVII. SKIPPING WITH THE HOOP.

The *exercises with a hoop*, are not as various and exercising as those with the short rope; they deserve, however, to be practised, and this is done on the same place where the exercises with the short rope are performed.

The hoop must be firmly joined at the ends, without knots, of such a diameter as to reach to the hips of the pupil using it.

The hoop is not firmly taken hold of with the hands, because it is put into a revolving motion, not by means of the hands, but of swinging (see pl. VI, fig. 10).

I. Skipping over the hoop from before. In this exercise, and in the two following (II, and III), the hoop is held with both hands, some inches from each other, before the body. The hoop passes first under the feet, and then over the head.

II. Skipping over the hoop from behind. The hoop passes first over the head, and then under the feet.

III. Skipping with a run:

a. gallopping; after each skipping, both feet touch the ground, but always the same foot first;

b. trotting; after each skipping, one foot only touches the ground, while the other is raised.

IV. Skipping from the side, with half a revolution of the hoop. One hand raises the hoop, and swings it through under the feet, and, after a spring, back. With the right, and left hand.

V. Skipping from the side with an entire revolution of the hoop. The same mode of taking hold of the hoop as in the preceding exercise, but the hoop, after having passed under the feet, continues its revolution over the head;

a. the hoop passing first under the feet, then over the head (from without to within);

b. the hoop passing first over the head, and then under the feet (from within to without).

XVIII. SKIPPING WITH THE ROPE.

A. With the short rope, swung by the pupil himself.

The rope should be from 1-2 to 3-4 of an inch thick, and so long, as to reach to the hips, on both sides, when the pupil stands upon it. For cross-skipping, it must be a little longer.

The carriage in this exercise, as well as in the preceding, is that for the preparatory exercises, page 1.

The arms, bent a little, are brought near to the body; the hands near the hips, stretched forth a little,

the swinging of the rope is performed merely by turning the wrist-joints; the arms should move either not at all, or but very little.

I. Simple skipping.
   a. Straight skipping,
     on the spot,
       from before,
       from behind;
     with running,
       galloping,
       trotting.

   b. Crossed skipping, wherein the lower arms are crossed;
     1. with the same crossing:
       on the spot:
         from before,
         from behind;
       with running:
         galloping,
         trotting;
     2. with changed crossing, one time the right arm over the left, the next time, the left over the right, and so on;
       on the spot:

from before,
from behind;
with running:
galloping,
trotting.

II. Double skipping, wherein the rope, at every spring, passes twice under the feet.

 a. Strait skipping.
 b. Crossed skipping.

In both kinds (*a* and *b*), the same variations as above, under I.

III. Turning, in order to change the skipping from before into that from behind, and the reverse.

 a. The pupil swings the rope, the moment when he ought to pass it from before to behind under the feet, by his right side upwards, turns himself swiftly right, and skips from behind to before.

This is to be performed also with turning to the left.

 b. The pupil turns the moment he has passed the rope from behind forwards under the feet, and skips from before backwards.

This should be done at first slowly, gradually as quick and long as possible.

In practising the crossed and double kinds of skipping, it is well to render it easier by changing with the simple. In general it is a beautiful exercise, to change in a certain order with the different kinds of skipping.

All the different kinds of skipping may be performed, the knees being stretched or bent, touching the breech with the heels, hopping on one foot, or changing the foot at every spring.

 B. With the long rope, swung by another person.

The rope should be 3-4 of an inch thick, soft and flexible, and from 16 to 20 feet long. The rope is fastened to a post, about three feet and a half above the ground. He who swings the rope, takes hold of it about 14 feet from where it is fastened, and gives it an elliptical motion; this is done by a slight turning of the hand, so that the axis of the ellipsis, described by the rope, is changed as little as possible; the rope should pass close over the ground. Some dexterity in swinging the rope quickly or slowly, as well as in following the motion of the pupil, is soon acquired.

The exercises with the long rope are thus divided:

I. where the pupil remains on the spot. The pupil stands forwards, backwards, or sideways to the middle of the rope which, according to this position, is swung from before, from behind, or from the side, under the feet. The knees are either stretched, or bent, or the breech struck with the heels at every spring;

II. where the pupil does not remain on the spot:

a. running through. The rope is turned off from the pupil. The moment the rope is rising, before his knees, the pupil runs behind the rope which going up affords time for his running off. This can be exercised by a whole line, one after the other;

b. leaping over the rope. The rope is turned towards the pupil. The moment when it, in coming down, is before his eyes, he makes the spring, after which he must quickly run off, not to be caught by the rope;

c. jumping to the rope, and running off. The same motion of the rope, the pupil improves the proper moment, approaches the rope, and begins skipping; after some revolutions of the rope, he runs off as in the preceding exercise, or backwards;

d. the same exercise, except that the pupil skips only once, and runs off, without waiting a second revolution of the rope;

e. skipping in a single line (*a*, and *b*). The number is so large as to form a circle, the centre of which is the post, and the semi-diameter half the length of the rope. The running is continually going on, and with each revolution of the rope, one runs through (*a*), or skips (*b*).

On the other side of the post another rope can be in motion, moving in the same, or an opposite direction, so that each one has, in each circuit, to run through, or skip over two ropes; or run through one, and skip over the other;

f. skipping in a double line. Two lines in a direction opposite to each other, one runs under, the other skips over, the rope or ropes.

All these exercises with the long rope can be combined with those with the short rope, and hoop, and a large number of variations and combinations made.

APPENDIX.

A NUMBER OF SINGLE EXERCISES.

I. Passing one or both legs over a short rod, or staff, held by the hands, or over the hands themselves, joined;
    a. one leg,
       1. the foot of the other leg standing,
       2. hopping on one leg, and passing the same over;
    both kinds are to be practised
       with the right, and left leg;
       forwards, and backwards;
    b. both legs at a time,
       only hopping,
          forwards and backwards.

II. Entire turning around one's own axis in a jump, on the spot, to the right, and left.

III. Sitting down, and rising, without the use of the hands:
    a. the legs bent, and crossed;
    b. one leg stretched forth which should not touch the ground in sitting down, or rising; on one foot, therefore: It is to be practised right and left;
    c. lying down, the arms crossed, and rising without the assistance of the arms and hands. This can be practised by a whole line at a time, to see who gets up first.

IV. Taking hold of the ear, and passing through the arm:

 a. with the left hand the right ear, and the right arm passing through;

 b. with the right hand the left ear, and the left arm passing through.

The ear can be taken hold of:

 1. at the upper part, which is easier,

 2. at the ear-lap, which is more difficult.

V. Touching the forehead with the foot. Placing the foot upon the neck. Both exercises are to be practised right and left.

VI. Slinging the arm, and hand around the occiput, so far as to reach with the points of the fingers to the chin, or further; right and left.

VII. Drawing out a knife, stuck in the ground near to the little toe, the hand of the opposite side passing around behind the feet which are standing fast, and straight out; right and left.

VIII. Taking up some object from the ground before, the heels being but a few inches from a wall.

IX. Touching the ground with the fingers, the knees being kept stiff.

X. Taking up a coin, or something like it, with the mouth from the earth, at a distance little less than one's own length, without touching the ground with the body.

XI. The right hand takes hold of the left ear-lap, the left of a piece of wood in the shape of a plate; this arm is stretched, and the body inclined forwards so far, as to touch the earth with the plate. Then after having turned around three times in this position, the body is raised, the ear-lap let loose, the arm with the plate held horizontally, and an experiment made to walk straight forward.

XII. A couple, equally tall and heavy, stand on a level ground, facing each other, toes touching toes; arms and hands are stretched, the latter hooking; the upper part of the body inclines backwards; in this position the couple revolves, to the right or left, without loosening their grasp.

These two exercises, XI, and XII, are very good means, to prevent dizziness.

XIII. Leaning against a wall in a straight position, the feet removing gradually from the wall, and pushing off the head from the wall, the elastic power proceeding from the back and neck, the arms kept straight, and close to the body.

XIV. Sitting on a ball, jug, or something like it; the legs are stretched out forwards, so that one heel only touches the ground.

Another mode is, to cross the legs over a stick which is resting with one end on the earth, with the other on the legs.

In either of these positions different things are to be done which require some moving, without losing the balance.

XV. Bending the joints of the wrist, the fingers being interlaced, and the elbows pressed against one another. The pressure is continued only until the joints of the wrists, not of the fingers, bend. It may be exercised :

  a. with one hand :
    left against left,
    left against right,
    right against right.
  b. with both hands,
  the right hand of one person interlaces with the left of the other.

Two onsets are made that each one may once have the advantage of having his thumb on the outside.

XVI. Tests for the strength of the arms :

  a. Stretching, and bending arms. One stretches out his arm, keeping it as stiff as possible, the fist firmly clenched. The other takes hold of the arm above the wrist from without, with the hand opposite to the stretched arm; if one stretches out his right arm, the other takes hold with his left hand. He who endeavors to bend, stands on the outside of the stretched arm; he places his other hand over that of the stretched arm, so that the same fingers rest upon one another, and the thumb crosses the thumb. He endeavors in this position to bend the joint of the wrist of the first by a strong pressure upon the fist, and a firm hold upon the wrist ; as soon as the wrist is bent, the elbow yields.

The bending must be brought on by an uniform pressure.

b. Two sit down at a narrow table, both resting the same elbow on it, so that the lower arm and hand incline forwards. Both join their hands, and endeavor, by an uniform pressure, to press down the other's arm. The other hand remains under the table, and rests on the thigh. It is to be exercised

  left against left,

  right against right.

XVII. The wrists are placed on the sides, so that the elbows form sharp angles ; the elbows are moved forwards, until they touch, then backwards.

XVIII. Two stand with their backs against each other, hook their arms, and lift each other in turns.

XIX. Moving along on the hands :

a. when sitting on the earth, the arms are stretched, so that they raise the body to a suspended position, and then move along, the legs being kept straight. The movement is made

  forwards,

  backwards, and

  to either side.

b. From the position of crouching described among the preparatory exercises (see page 3, V, *a*; pl. I, fig. 3). The hands are, the arms between the knees, placed upon the earth, the knees pressing against them, the body rests in a suspended position, and moves along upon the arms,

  forwards,

  backwards, and

  to either side.

XX. Jump against the wall; the right foot steps over the left, placed against the wall, and the body turns, in descending, towards the left. The same is to be done to the right.

XXI. Running up a wall; the body turns in descending. It is well to have a board which is at first put up in a slanting position, the angle of its inclination gradually increasing to a right.

XXII. Winding with a staff. The hands take hold of the staff as in leaping with a pole, described above, (page 17, pl. II, fig. 2), and put it firmly against the ground. If the right hand is up, the left foot stands forth. The pupil passes with his body, inclined backwards, under the staff, and back again. The lower the grasp, the more difficult the exercise.

XXIII. Stepping over the staff. The staff is thin, and about three feet long.

a. First kind:

1. The hands take hold of the staff behind the back, the thumbs turned outwards;
2. the staff is raised over the head, and lowered before the body;
3. stepping over with one foot after the other;
4. returning with the staff.

b. Second kind:

1. the same as *a*, 1;
2. the same as *a*, 2;
3. one foot, the right or left, winds around one arm and steps over;
4. the other hand raises the staff over the head;
5. stepping back with the same foot;
6. raising the staff over the head to its first position.

XXIV. Stepping through.

a. Both hands are placed flat on the fore-corners of a chair, the arms being kept stiff; one foot steps through first, and, as soon as it has reached the ground, the other.

The hands are not allowed to be lifted, and the seat of the chair must not be touched at all, or, at most, very slightly, with the sole. The pupil can begin and end,
1. standing on the left side of the chair,
2. on the right.

 b. One hand rests flat on one fore-corner, the other, in a diagonal direction, on the hind-corner:
1. left hand on the fore-corner,
2. right hand on the fore-corner.

XXV. Throwing the right leg forwards, with a jerk, as in the act of kicking, then the left, alternately.

XXVI. The right hand takes hold of the left foot, the right leg is bent, until the body reaches the ground, then stretched again. The same is to be done with the left leg.

XXVII. The right arm is stretched forwards, in a horizontal direction, the right leg is raised, until it touches the right arm. The same is to be done with the left arm and leg.

XXVIII. A round pole, four feet long, three inches thick, rests on two posts, four or five feet above the ground. A peg, two inches long, is put in a hole on the side of the pole towards the ground. A rope, 15 or 20 feet long, and 1-2 or 3-4 of an inch thick, is thrown over the pole so that the two ends hang down on the same side. The gymnick, on the side where the ends hang, places his right foot in the bow formed by the hanging rope on the other side, takes hold of the ends, passes his left foot through between the rope, and with it knocks the peg out of its place ; then draws the left leg back, and lowers himself to the ground. However easy this exercise is, falling down is frequent, and, on this account, the pole ought not to be higher than mentioned above, and the earth below to be soft.

SECOND SECTION.

GYMNASTICK GAMES.

OF GYMNASTICK GAMES IN GENERAL.

The *gymnastick games* form an essential part of gymnasticks, and, therefore, every gymnastick institution should have a large place, without the precincts of the gymnasium, destined for this purpose, and consisting of high-grown wood, thickets, bushes, and bare spaces.

There is, in every place, a number of plays common, but not all, usually played, can be recommended, or at least they are not equally useful as others. Our object, therefore, will be not so much to describe new plays, but to shew what renders some superior to others.

In the first place, all games which are played sitting, however useful in other respects, are to be exempted; a good gymnastick play requires motion, in order to attain its end, which is, to render the body active and strong.

In the second place all plays for gain are excluded; youths are to vie for superiority in dexterity and strength, not for pecuniary advantage; this passion discovers itself soon enough in man, and cannot be counteracted too early.

A good gymnastick play should not require too great and extensive preparations;

it should be easy to be understood, and yet founded on a certain rule and principle;

it should not entirely, or to a great extent, depend on chance;

it should occupy a sufficiently large number;

it should not require too large a space unproportioned to the number of players;

it should not require idle lookers on; but, contrary, each one should be occupied;

it should afford a fair proportion of labor and rest;

it should not be uniform and without variety;

it should require active and dexterous players, in order to be played well;

it should be of such a nature as to be always played with zeal and interest.

DESCRIPTION OF SOME GAMES.

A. Games which may be played in the gymnasium itself.

I. The number of players, not under 20 nor above 100, are standing on one side of the place destined for playing. One is chosen who, distinguished by some mark, takes his place on the opposite side. He asking: *are you afraid of your enemy?* advances, and the others, answering with *no!* start from their goal, endeavoring to reach the opposite side without being caught. On the other hand the single one strives to catch as many as possible, before they reach the opposite side. He who is caught and receives three claps in succession by the single one, is of his party and catches, beginning from the following run. When all who have not been caught, have reached the opposite side, the single one, with his prisoners, takes the other side, so that both have changed sides. Then the same course is repeated, with the exception that all who have been lawfully made prisoners in the preceding run, have the right to catch. Thus the play is continued till all are taken.

If, at last, a small number, or only one, have run three times without being taken, they or he are free and victors.

Those who catch, must always start at a time from their goal. If one of the other party is found on the side which his party has just left, he is to be considered a prisoner, though he has not been struck; and likewise he who passes over the limit on the right or left side. Each one as soon as he is taken, must put on a mark.

II. The whole number of players, not under 20 nor above 60, arrange themselves in pairs according to their dexterity in running. Of these pairs two parties are formed of equal number, each of which take one side. One of the parties send one to challenge who, stopping a few paces from the opposite side, selects one of the hostile party. Both stand touching each other with the right foot; the challenged leans forwards without raising the left foot; the challenger leans backwards, strikes the other, with one hand, three times, as quick or slowly as he pleases, upon one or both hands, and, after the third stroke, takes to his heels. The challenged endeavors to strike him immediately after the third stroke, or in pursuing. If he succeeds, the challenger is prisoner. If not, before the middle of the ground, then the challenging party sends another out, before whom the challenged must retreat.

In general the ruling principle of the play is that every one must yield to, or can be taken prisoner, receiving a stroke, by any one of the opposite party who has started later from the goal. Although starting may not be done in a certain order, yet in most cases it should be considered as a rule, that each one runs only against one whose equal he is in running. Care must be taken lest some run too seldom, others too often, sometimes too many at a time, or none at all. The play must go on uniformly, and all the players ought to be equally occupied.

Three or four paces distant from each goal, on the same side (always in the diagonal corners of the place), a post, or something of the kind, is fixed at which the prisoners are placed. These are standing with legs straddling as far as they can conveniently, touching one another with their feet. The farthest (the nearest his own party) stretches his arm towards his party. Each party may free their prisoners; only the farthest requires to be touched, and all are ransomed who stood touching each other; yet the liberator must take heed not to be struck, before he has achieved his object.

Ransoming imparts a great deal of life into the game, each party endeavoring to redeem their friends taken, and watching the adversaries in their power. It is evident that the difficulty of the latter increases with the number of prisoners.

Laws of the play:

1. From four to six prisoners, according to the number of the players, make a play.
2. The party gaining, challenges in the next play.
3. As soon as one is taken prisoner, the play stops until each party is at their goal, and the prisoner in his place.
4. He who passes over the limits, on the right or left, is prisoner.
5. Players can leave only at the termination of a play.
6. At the same time new players may be received, as long as the number of sixty is not exceeded.

B. Games which are to be played without the precincts of the gymnasium.

A place of the following description is most suitable for some of these plays.

A woody place from 200 to 400 paces square. Young pines, and thick underwood, which are intersected by some bare places, small hills, and dales, or ditches, are best. The number of the players should be distributed in such a manner as to leave, after the necessary garrisons are taken off, an equal number on both sides. The one party has four castles, each about 20 to 50 paces distant from a corner of the place; the other party a town in the centre.

The garrison of the town should consist at least of two men, and always be as strong as those of two castles together. If there are from 50 to 60 players, four are to be garrisoned in the town, two in each of the castles.

The object of the whole play is now, by making prisoners, to weaken the enemy so as to disable them to resist in open field and battle. The necessary combats are done in wrestling. The leaders should take care, lest it degenerates into a mere scuffle. Striking and boxing is unlawful. In order to succeed in the latter object, it is necessary to observe the following rules.

An open battle should be avoided, unless its successful issue is sure. The enemy ought to be drawn from their fortified places towards those of the adversary. Small detachments or individuals should be sent out, to ascertain the enemy's position, strength of their garrisons, places where they keep the prisoners; single posts or sentinels should be cut off, and arrested; from hiding places and ambuscades damage should be done to the enemy, false attacks and surprises performed. The most violent struggle arises in taking and redeeming prisoners. Only gymnicks well skilled and experienced in wrestling, should be admitted to this play; nor should there be a mixture of very different ages. If those of 16 and 17 years play, none of 12 and 13 should be admitted.

The most important laws of the play are:

1. There are four castles and one town.
2. The players are distributed so as to leave an equal number after the places have been garrisoned.
3. The garrison of the town must be equal to those of two castles.
4. If the garrison is complete, no place can be taken; if not, the place can be taken by a force, five times greater than the garrison.
5. Deserted places are taken and garrisoned with the number fixed for them.
6. One man as guard is requisite for every two prisoners.
7. Prisoners are freed, if the succor is five times stronger than the guards.

8. Prisoners are freed at any rate, if the enemy, with their whole remaining force (which, however, must be superior to the number of prisoners) appears before the place, when only the fixed garrison is in it.

If the number of players is considerably less, they should play with only two castles situated opposite each other in a diagonal line.

II. The same place, described in the preceding play is suitable for this too; and if such an one should not be obtained, one of 100 paces long and 50 broad, will be sufficient.

One of the players is chosen hunter, who selects for himself, according to the size of the place, from one to three companions. Hunter and his companions should wear some conspicuous mark. The game assemble in the place where they are free from pursuit. The hunter having called: *free departure!* all the game disperse, and conceal themselves in the woods. After some time the hunter, having cried out: *free departure at an end!* sets out on his pursuit, with his companions. From this moment the game is allowed to return to the refuge, provided they escape the hunter and his companions. The latter have only the right of seizing the game, but this is not considered really taken, before the hunter has given three claps. He who is taken in this way, becomes one of the hunter's companions: and, in the next chase, assists in pursuing and seizing. The hunter, finding no more game in the wood, after his return to the refuge, cries again: *free departure at an end*, and thus the play continues, till all are taken.

If at last a few, or only one, have been three times hunted without being caught, they are considered free.

III. It is very well to have some mounds or elevations 20 feet and more high, steep but of a soft loose earth. According to the equal extent of these elevations the gymnicks are divided into parties; each party starts upon a word or signal; he who reaches the top first, has gained.

The number may be divided into two bodies, one of which takes possession of the top, the other ascends the mound in storm. Whoever of the aggressors is dragged up, or, when running up, falls, or is thrown down, is prisoner; whoever of the defendants is drawn down, is likewise prisoner, and neither of them is allowed to continue his part in the play. The exhaustion of either party terminates the play.

IV. Playing ball is very much to be commended, since it, however simple, unites various exercises: throwing, striking, running, catching, etc. The play in its principle is too well known, in all parts of the couutry, to require any description, or explanation. The many variations in different parts, are altogether unessential, and matter of choice.

THIRD SECTION.

MANAGEMENT OF A GYMNASIUM.

MANAGEMENT OF A GYMNASIUM.

GYMNASTICK EXERCISES are intended to restore the just proportion of the two principal parts of human education, moral and physical, the latter of which had been neglected for the space of several ages. As long as man has a body, it is his duty to take care of, to cultivate it, as well as his mind, and consequently gymnastick exercises should form an essential part of education. Where man exists, there gymnastick exercises have, or at least ought to have, a place; they are the property of mankind, not confined to any one nation, or part of a nation. It is true, this art, as well as all other institutions belonging to mankind, will assume a different form in different regions; climate, locality, state of civilization, manners in general, form of government, religion will exercise their influence in producing a different form, but the essence remains the same, culture of the body.

It is not our object to stand up as advocates for gymnastick exercises; we take it for granted, that they are not only a useful, but necessary part of education. Every village, however insignificant, ought to, and could, have a gymnasium, as well as institutions for mental education. One completely furnished gymnasium, at least, ought to be in every county. National days might be proper occasions for the youth of the country to shew to their parents the progress they have made in dexterity and strength. The day when the counsellors of the country declared its independence, the days, when the defenders of the country bought that blessing with their heart's blood, might be proper occasions to shew to the nation that her sons are able to preserve what their fathers have obtained.

In order to illustrate the subject for which this section is destined, management of a gymnasium, we shall treat of the following parts separately.

1. OF THE INSTRUCTOR IN GYMNASTICKS.

The instructor in gymnasticks has, of all instructors, the most difficult situation. The business of other teachers, is to teach a certain science, in which they, by their daily occupation, almost necessarily advance. The instructor in gymnasticks ought not only to know but also to perform what he teaches. The teacher of a science will always be in advance of his scholars, but the instructor of gymnasticks will soon be equalled by most, and surpassed by some of his pupils. He ought, nevertheless, to be always intent on obtaining as much dexterity in the different exercises, as his bodily constitution allows. Self practice and experience alone afford a clear and distinct idea of every movement and exercise, and of the effects which each one produces. He should carefully avoid becoming ridiculous to the younger boys on account of striking awkwardness and indexterity: The older pupils, for the most part, are satisfied with good intention, and laborious experiment. Even if he is wanting in dexterity in single exercises, yet he should be perfectly acquainted with all parts of gymnasticks, and be familiar with the principles of all. The pupils must be enabled to respect him as a man of education; else he appears, in spite of all dexterity and skill, as a mere juggler.

An instructor in gymnasticks ought strictly to observe the following laws:

1. not to give a bad example, either in, or out of the gymnasium;

2. to refrain, during the time destined for exercises, from all those enjoyments and gratifications which are improper for youth, as smoking or chewing tobacco, drinking spirits, etc.;

3. not to appear too late in the gymnasium, but to be there with the first;

4. to observe himself all laws which have been found necessary, most strictly, and to be the severest judge against himself;

5. not to endeavor to outdo his pupils, but to practise quietly and modestly, without any noise and ostentation.

6. to direct the conversation of the pupils so that it may be instructive and entertaining, and not offensive in word or thought;

7. to avoid all stiffness and pedantry, and to be friendly and kind, without surrendering the necessary respect;

8. to prove clearly that he is impressed with the importance of the subject, and not induced by mercenary motives, and vanity;

9. to understand how to deal with his pupils, that they may love and respect him as a man;

10. to act as an elder friend, adviser, and warner among his pupils.

II. OF THE EXERCISES.

All exercise has its law and rule, method and discipline, measure and end. In gymnastick exercises one thing follows from the other; the single exercises supply and complete each other, and must be practised by turns. While some members rest after labor, others may exercise; no partiality should be allowed as to right and left. The object is to exercise the limbs, not to perform a feat.

There are, indeed, exercises which must be necessarily practised one after the other; but many must be practised at the same time, else the sameness, even of the most useful exercise, will injure the formation and culture of the body in general. If the greatest perfection in one exercise should be obtained before commencing another, the whole period of youth would not suffice to become perfect only in a few exercises.

Although a pupil should not be occupied constantly with the same exercise, yet there are some, with which the beginning should be made, and which form the introduction and preparation, as it were, for the whole of gymnastick exercises. Every boy, or youth, who has not exercised before, is either entirely stiff, or if he possesses some limberness, he rarely understands to execute a regular movement. The *preparatory exercises* (see page 1 to 7) remove these deficiencies most effectually. They must be practised by every new comer first and considerably, and afterwards frequently repeated. After this introduction the simplest part of every exercise should be commenced, viz: of *running* (see page 8), *leaping* (see page 11), *climbing* (see page 97), *drawing* (see page 117), *moving the body, resting on, or suspended by, the arms,* along the *single bar* (see page 66, IX), *moving the body, resting on the arms,* along the *parallel bars* (see page 87, VIII), and *balancing* (see page 48). In this way the strength of each one is easily ascertained, and how the deficiencies may be remedied.

In the beginning, especially when a new gymnasium is at once completely furnished, it is well to establish as a rule, that the gymnicks practice only such exercises, as have been particularly shewn to them. Being unexperienced, they might easily injure themselves, if, left to themselves, they would try new exercises.

As soon as some progress has been made *in a gymnasium*, the instructor should choose, or cause to be chosen, monitors from the most sensible and dexterous. The monitors should instruct the new comers in the preparatory exercises, and perform themselves, whenever it is necessary. They must understand how to assist in performing a movement, be especially attentive to avoid an injury, where sliding or falling is possible. They must be able to make a judicious selection from the single parts of a compound exercise. In inspecting the younger and weaker, they should consider that the object is general preparation for gymnastick exercises, not performing particular exercises or feats.

III. OF THE TIME FOR EXERCISES.

The problem, to occupy many gymnicks at the same time, is to be solved in a gymnasium. The time, allotted to exercises, should not be too short. Two afternoons, or the larger part of them, in a week, would certainly not be too much to spend in this important part of education. If the time is too short, many are apt to exert themselves too much, and thus to injure, rather than benefit themselves.

The whole time is divided into two portions, the first of which is destined for exercises which each one selects according to his inclination; the second for the regular instruction. During the former, every one chooses his occupation, and practises those exercises, which he likes best, or in which he perceives himself deficient, or which he wishes particularly to cultivate. But both, the instructor and monitors, should be always about, to preserve order, or to direct now this one, now that one. During this voluntary occupation, the instructor has the best opportunity to observe the inclination, talents, exertions, development, progress, and dexterity of every one.

At the expiration of this time, the gymnicks assemble, and, after some rest, satisfy their hunger and thirst with some bread and water. All the pupils are, once for all, distributed into classes, according to age or size. If there should be some considerably stronger or weaker, so as to create inconvenience in exercising with those of the same size or age, they should be put in the next older or younger class.

Here we should advise to keep the most accurate account of each individual as to his frequenting the gymnasium, and industry while there. Since the introduction of gymnastick exercises is so new, and by no means tested so much as might be desirable, it is well that the inferences, drawn from observation, should be founded upon certain facts, not vague suppositions. The duty towards the public, and the cause of physical education, demands such an accuracy, and it occasions but little trouble.

All the exercises are divided into as many classes as there are classes of gymnicks, and are shifted every day, so that in a series of days every pupil passes through all classes of exercises. A monitor is appointed for every class.

IV. OF THE DRESS.

A dress for gymnastick exercises should be durable, cheap, and fit for all movements. Linen, not yet bleached, is the best material; and a jacket, or round-about, and pantaloons, the best form. If the changing dresses of fashion are worn, they will affect the exercises, and then these must be divided into exercises for rich, and poor.

All exercises are performed with head and hands bare.

Cravats and neckcloths of all descriptions, but especially those which prevent the free movements of the head and neck, are not only inconvenient, but injurious.

Suspenders should not impede the expansion of the chest, therefore never have any cross-pieces passing, in any direction, over the breast.

Boots should not be too high and heavy, but allow a free use of the joints of the foot.

Pantaloons ought to be made so that they allow a free use of the lower extremities; it is injurious both to health and freedom of motion, to have them fastened, around the waist, with a girdle or belt; they should hang merely by the suspenders. Equally inconvenient, if not injurious, are straps, fastening the pantaloons around the feet.

During exercising, the dress can scarcely be too light and cool; after exercising, a coat is of service to prevent taking cold. On this account, a frock-coat is better than any other, because it defends not only the back, but the front, most susceptible of cold.

V. OF THE RESTING-PLACE.

During exercising nothing should be spoken, except what concerns the exercise. But, then, there should be a place for rest and conversation. This place should be shaded by trees, and provided with benches, and a black board for the necessary advertisements and communications.

VI. OF THE SPECTATORS.

A gymnasium is no theatre, and no one has a right to expect a spectacle. But on the other hand a gymnasium is no secret abode, though it must have its fixed precincts separating the gymnick from the mere spectator. The places for the single exercises should be arranged in such a manner as to afford a perfect view for those without the precincts. Thus every man has an opportunity to obtain a correct idea of the character and value of gymnastick exercises.

The parents, instructers, and guardians of the children, have a good opportunity to observe their children, pupils, and wards, left to themselves among their equals. In this way they are enabled to look deeper into the dispositions and peculiarities of their young friends, than if they kept them constantly by themselves. Thus the whole publick discharges the office of overseers of morals.

VII. OF THE LAWS.

Good manners and morals must rule in a gymnasium with a more powerful sway, than elsewhere strict laws. The greatest punishment which can be inflicted, is exclusion from the gymnastick community.

A. General laws.

1. Every one who desires to become a pupil in a gymnasium, must promise that he will observe the necessary laws and arrangements.

2. No one shall show a sentiment of hostility which he may entertain against any one of the gymnicks, during the season of exercise, but each shall exercise in peace and cheerfulness.

3. Every gymnick shall exercise only with coat, hat, and neckcloth laid aside.

4. Every gymnick shall exercise in his turn, as he arrives at the place of a single exercise.

5. The gymnicks divide themselves into parties for the single exercises.

6. The number, fixed for each party, shall not be exceeded.

7. No one shall go from one party to another, except the exercises of the former should be too difficult.

8. No one shall intrude into a party when complete, but wait, till one resigns his place, or the whole party stops.

9. The number for the single parties is as follows:

In throwing, not over 12.
In leaping without a pole, not over 12.
In leaping with a pole, not over 8.
In leaping over the ditch without a pole, not over 20.
In leaping over a ditch with a pole, not over 12.
In vaulting, not over 10.
On the single bar, not over 8.
On the parallel bars, not over 8.
In balancing, not over 12.
In skipping with the long rope, not over 12.

10. Every one shall keep from that side near an instrument, from which the start is made.

11. Every one shall make use only of the instruments and utensils in exercises for which each is destined, and on the place appropriate for each exercise. All moveable instruments (as lances, poles for leaping, etc.) must be returned to their place, after they have been used.

12. During exercising nothing shall be spoken, except what concerns the exercise.

13. He who wishes to look at some exercise, can stand, sit, or lie at a proper distance from the instrument.

14. The exercise should never be covered, or concealed towards the bounds by persons standing before.

B. Special laws.

a. For running.

15. There shall be no talking during running, especially during the racing of many.

16. After running none shall stand still, or sit, or lie, but walk about, in order to cool, and refresh himself by degrees.

b. For leaping.

17. The stands for leaping with and without a pole, as well as the strings and pegs belonging to each stand, shall not be confounded.

18. There shall be no pulling, pushing, or climbing up the posts or stands. Two persons shall raise the pegs, improving one or two steps, fixed to the stands for this purpose.

19. The poles to be used are of a length from 7 to 11 feet, and of a proportionate thickness. If any one keeps his own pole, he shall conform with these measures, and mark the pole with his name. Other poles shall be removed.

20. No one shall make use of poles not his own. He who has none of his own, shall use those belonging to the gymnasium.

21. He is not yet qualified for leaping with a pole, to whom a pole of seven feet, and a proportionate thickness, is too heavy.

c. For vaulting.

22. No one shall practise vaults, before he has attained some dexterity in the preparatory exercises.

23. Those who wish to join particular classes for vaulting, shall be able to fulfil the following conditions :

    a. to climb up a rope to the height of 40 feet ;

b. to perform the principal exercises on the single bar;

c. to perform the principal exercises on the parallel bars;

d. to leap without a pole to the height of his own hips;

e. to perform all the preparatory exercises with considerable dexterity.

d. For balancing.

24. The balancing-pole shall be ascended only on the thick end.

25. In a balancing-combat, only three shall be standing on the balancing-pole, the two engaged in the middle, a third waiting on the thick end.

26. In balancing, only three shall be on the pole; two balancing, and one waiting. As soon as the first draws near the thin end, the second shall stand still.

27. As each one alights from the balancing-pole, he must stop its vibrations.

28. All joggling and tossing on the balancing-pole, is forbidden; nor shall any one pass beneath the balancing-pole, while any person is exercising.

e. For the single bar.

29. No one shall exercise at a bar, which he is unable to reach standing, or by means of a jump.

f. For the parallel bars.

30. No one shall exercise on bars on which he cannot come to rest upon his arms, by means of hopping.

31. All standers by shall keep at some distance from the bars on all sides.

g. For climbing.

32. The ropes shall not be used for any kind of swinging.

33. When some one is climbing, no one shall hinder him, whether by following, or stretching the rope, unless the climber desire it.

34. No one is allowed to ascend the ladder of a climbing-instrument, unless he be able to climb up the rope belonging to the same instrument.

35. Only on a very high rope the climber is allowed to descend on the ladder; on other ropes he shall descend by the rope, or climbing-pole.

36. Only two are allowed to be on the top of a climbing-instrument, and the first must come down as soon as a third begins to climb up.

37. Only one shall sit upon the cross of the climbing-poles, and only so long, as is necessary to gain strength.

38. No one shall practise on a rope, if he cannot climb up the next lowest one.

39. No one shall be standing within the climbing-instruments.

h. For throwing with lances.

40. Every one shall use the lances, belonging to the gymnasium, or his own, marked with his name, not those of others.

41. The measures for lances are: six, seven, or eight feet long, 1, 1 1-4, or 1 1-2 inches thick. No lance of a different measure shall be used.

i. For throwing with balls.

42. No one shall leave a ball on the ground, but put it in the box.

43. The ground destined for this exercise shall not be approached by lookers on, or at least only from the back of those exercising.

j. For wrestling.

44. No one shall refuse a challenge for wrestling, unless when unwell, tired, or prevented by some evil; dress shall not be an excuse.

k. For games.

45. All who are too small or weak, or have not yet passed through the preparatory exercises, shall be excluded from the gymnastick plays.

46. No one shall join a party of players, unless he was present at the distribution.

47. A general agreement of the party playing, can make an exception from the established rules of a play.

FOURTH SECTION.

OF THE FOUNDATION AND ARRANGE-
MENT OF A GYMNASIUM.

OF THE FOUNDATION AND ARRANGEMENT OF A GYMNASIUM.

Directions for founding and arranging a gymnasium, cannot be given so as to be suitable for all single cases. Much depends on locality, circumstances, and wants. Such particularities cannot be regarded, but only the general principles which are to be observed in any given case. To illustrate these principles by example, the enumeration of the instruments for several gymnasiums of a different rate will be added.

I. *Of the situation of a gymnasium.*

If a gymnasium is to be founded for a public school or institution, where gymnasticks form a part of the daily regular instruction, a place in the vicinity would be necessary, yet a public place in a city would not be desirable for various reasons. But if a gymnasium is intended for one or several villages, a whole town, or a remote institution, where the free afternoons can be appropriated to gymnastick exercises, there is no objection to having the place at a distance of one or two miles. For children of eight and nine years, whose age does not allow of a continued occupation, have an excellent exercise in taking such a walk.

It is desirable that every gymnasium should possess the following qualities; a level, but high situation (for on an elevated place, the air is better, nor are the exercises interrupted so frequently by wet and dampness); firm soil, covered with turf, and grown with trees (but not with pines of any description; for their leaves, fruit, and roots only occasion slipping and falling); oaks, elms, maples, and, where they are common, lindens, are the most suitable trees. If trees are altogether wanting, some should be planted, at least around the boundaries, the place for rest, and between the grounds for the single exercises, so that the trees might answer the purposes of limits, marks, and shade. The trees, if they are high, may serve to fix a part of the climbing apparatus on them, and thus save a part of the greatest expense of furnishing a gymnasium. It is well to select a situation, little or not at all exposed to the north and east winds. If a woody place borders on the gymnasium, suitable for plays, it is a great advantage.

If three and more hours are devoted to gymnastick exercises, there should be an opportunity of bringing water to the place without much trouble.

A principal want for a gymnasium which is at a distance from houses, is a building, which can be locked, for keeping the moveable apparatus. If the larger pieces, as ladders, are to be taken off in winter, then the building must have a length of 40 feet.

Where nature has done little, more must be done by labor and expense. If the soil is not pretty firm, the roads for leaping, vaulting, etc. ought to be covered with clay, stamped, and strewn with sand. If the soil of the race-ground is moist and rich, sand must be brought upon it. Tan, too, is very serviceable.

II. *Of the shape of a gymnasium.*

The most convenient shape of a gymnasium, is that of a parallelogram, the length of which is nearly the double of its width. Then the necessary extent can be given to the race-ground, nor is any exercise, on account of too great breadth of the place, covered by others to the spectators, without the precincts.

A gymnasium must have fixed boundaries, best a fence, at least a ditch. A fence with a hedge behind it, is a very good defence against large and small animals. A single or double row of trees around the gymnasium, adds greatly to its pleasantness.

A gymnasium requires an entry for foot passengers and vehicles. If the place destined for playing, lies towards another direction, one or two more entries are necessary. The roads from the entries to the place of rest, should not intersect the grounds of any exercises.

In selecting the grounds for the single exercises, care should be taken to bring those of the same kind together, as the grounds for running, leaping, etc. There should be an easy communication between the single places of exercise, so that it may not be necessary to cross one ground in order to come to another. Unless this is observed, a great confusion would arise, if most of the grounds are occupied, and one party changes their exercise. Order in this respect, cannot be carried too far. The roads of starting, belonging to the single exercises, as vaulting, leaping, should be marked as to their length and breadth. A ground grown with turf, facilitates it much; it only requires to cut out the turf. The limits between the single places for exercises, too, may easily be marked by small furrows.

It is well to have the place for rest, the barn, and the place to hang up the clothes, near together, and, if possible, in the centre of the gymnasium.

The moveable apparatus which should be brought into the barn every evening, is the following:

The apparatus for drawing.
The ropes for skipping.
The strings, bags, pegs, and poles for leaping.
The lances.
The saddle-cushions.
The balls.
The black-boards.

The ropes do not require to be taken off, but it is sufficient to draw them up, and sling them about the beams.

III. *Of the size of a gymnasium.*

Since the size of a gymnasium cannot be estimated otherwise, than by computing the size and number of the single places of exercises, we shall, once more, give a statement of the room requisite for every exercise, though it has already been done in describing the single exercises.

Room requisite:

for the race-ground, from 24 to 30 feet in width, from 300 to 400 in length (see page 8);

for the circles, 30 feet in width, 70 in length (see page 8);

for the stand for leaping without poles, 14 feet in width, 40 in length (see page 14);

for the stand for leaping with poles, 16 feet in width, 40 in length (see page 16);

for the ditch for leaping, 40 feet in width, 50 in length (see page 13);

for the steps for leaping, 20 feet in width, 40 in length (see page 16);

for the vaulting-bar, or horse, 20 feet in width, 40 in length (see page 19);

for the balancing-pole, from 12 to 16 feet in width, from 60 to 80 in length (see page 49);

for the single-bar, from 12 to 20 feet in width, from 16 to 20 in length (see page 57);

for the parallel bars, 12 feet in width, and 24 in length (see page 83);

for the instrument, described page 63, from 20 to 24 feet square;

for the instrument described page 99, 4, from 10 to 12 feet square;

for the climbing-instrument with one mast, 30 feet square (see page 98, 1);

for the climbing-instrument with two masts, 30 feet square (see page 99, 2);

for the climbing-instrument with four masts, 30 feet square (see page 99, 3);

for a climbing-pole, from 4 to 6 feet square (see page 97, 1);

for the ground for throwing with lances, 80 feet in width, 70 in length (see page 111);

for the ground for throwing with balls, first kind, 60 feet in width, from 120 to 140 in length (see page 113);

for the ground for throwing with balls, second kind, 30 feet in width, 40 in length (see page 115);

for the ground for drawing, from 10 to 12 feet in width, and if 20 on each side are to draw, at least 100 feet in length (see page 117);

for the ground for skipping with the long rope, a place of at least 30 feet diameter (see page 130);

for the ground for skipping with the short rope, from 20 to 30 feet in width, and about the same length; if the exercise is to be performed in running, the place requires a greater length (see page 129);

for the ground for preparatory exercises, at least 20 feet in width, and 40 in length (see page 1);

for the play-ground, from 60 to 120 feet in width, from 100 to 120 in length (see page 142);

for the place of rest, 50 feet square (see page 157);

for the barn and the place to hang up the clothes, 50 feet square (see page 167).

If it is ascertained how much apparatus is necessary, it is easy to compute the size of the place.

IV. *Of the apparatus of a gymnasium.*

The question is now to ascertain how much apparatus is requisite for a given number of pupils. *A gymnasium is to be considered completely furnished, only when all pupils can be occupied at the same time.*

According to the principle last mentioned, a *gymnasium for* 400 *pupils* requires a place 465 feet in length, and 260 in breadth, and the following apparatus and instruments:

1. *Race-ground.*
2. *Circles.*
3. Two long, and 30 short *ropes* for *skipping.*
4. A long, and a short *rope* for drawing; a *rope with neck-pieces*; *staves* for *drawing.*
5. Twelve *vaulting-bars*:
   a. with saddle-holds:
      1 three feet high;
      2 three feet 4 inches high;
      2 three feet 8 inches high;
      2 four feet high;
      1 four feet 4 inches high;
      1 four feet 8 inches high;
   b. without saddle-holds:
      1 three feet 6 inches high.
      1 four feet high.
      1 four feet 6 inches high.

The thickness, length, and proportion of the croup, saddle and neck may be seen in the following chapter.

6. Two *stands*, or two pair of posts for *leaping without poles.*
7. Three *stands*, or three pair of posts for *leaping with poles.*
8. A *ditch* for *leaping.*
9. *Steps* for *leaping down.*
10. Three *balancing-poles.*
11. Twelve *single bars*:
    2 three feet 6 inches high;
    2 four feet high;
    2 four feet 6 inches high;
    2 five feet high;
    1 five feet 6 inches high;
    1 six feet high;

1 six feet 6 inches high;
1 seven feet high;
12. Nine *parallel bars:*
1 two feet 6 inches high.
2 three feet high.
2 three feet 6 inches high.
2 four feet high.
1 four feet 6 inches high.
1 five feet high.

The proportional width may be seen in the following chapter.

13. *Climbing apparatus*
with one mast;
with two masts;
with four masts.

The last may be dispensed with, if the first two are what they ought to be.

Instrument for climbing by means of the arms alone, described page 99, 4;
three climbing-poles.

14. Instrument for moving in hanging, described page 63.
15. *Play-ground.*
16. *Ground* for *wrestling.*
17. *Ground* for *preparatory exercises.*
18. *Ground* for *throwing with balls*, first kind.
19. *Ground* for *throwing with balls*, second kind.
20. *Ground* for *throwing with darts.*

In a gymnasium for 200 pupils, the number of leaping-stands, vaulting, single, and parallel bars, would be considerably altered.

If the place is very limited, the play-ground is to be sought without the precincts of the gymnasium; the ground for throwing with balls, first kind, may be altogether given up; preparatory exercises and skipping with short ropes, may be practised on the race-ground. All this depends, however, on the locality. Where room is in abundan is better to take too much than too little.

All the calculations given above, are to be understood of a place not interrupted by trees, and similar objects.

. It is apparent from all that has been said, that still much is left to the judgment of him who arranges a gymnasium. It is of importance to have instruments in sufficient number and proper proportion, especially single, parallel, and vaulting-bars, and leaping-stands. The first two, and the last, are every where easily procured; if the vaulting-bars are too dear, a few may suffice, and vaulting be confined to the older pupils. A climbing-apparatus, always the most expensive part of a gymnasium, may be first dispensed with, provided that there are some high trees, to which several ropes and ladders may be attached.

It would be a great mistake to calculate that if the apparatus, enumerated above, is necessary for 400 pupils, 200 require one half, 100 one fourth, and 50 one eighth part of it. For 50 pupils of every age and size, require an apparatus of as many different degrees as 400, if not as many of each degree.

For those who have not yet been acquainted with gymnasticks, and would like to learn the principles according to which the apparatus is to be procured, we shall add one more example, that will, probably, answer the purpose, in many cases, where a gymnasium for a small community, is to be erected.

Necessary apparatus for eighty pupils.

1. Two *stands for leaping without poles.*

Two *stands for leaping with poles.* Both with strings, bags, and pegs.

Leaping-poles.

One *ditch for leaping.*

2. *Single bars*, four pieces:
   one, 3 feet 6 inches high;
   one, 4 feet 6 inches high;
   one, 5 feet 6 inches high;

one, 6 feet 6 inches high;
each 16 feet long.

3. *Parallel bars*, four pieces:
one 2 feet six inches high; 14 inches wide;
one 3 feet high; 15 inches wide;
one 3 feet 6 inches high; 16 inches wide;
one 4 feet 6 inches high; 18 inches wide;
each 8 feet long.

4. *Vaulting-bars*, four pieces, with saddle-holds:
one 3 feet high,
one 3 feet 4 inches high,
one 3 feet 8 inches high,
one 4 feet high.

5. One *balancing-pole*.

6. A *post for throwing with darts*, and *darts* at least for the older pupils.

7. One *rope for drawing* with the neck.
One *rope* from 20 to 30 feet long, and 3-4 of an inch thick, *for drawing*.

8. *Short ropes for skipping*, at least for the elder pupils.

9. *Ropes for climbing:*
one rope 20 feet long,
one rope 30 feet long;
both hung up in a manner as simple as possible.

10. *Climbing-poles:*
one from 20 to 30 feet high, and from 6 to 8 inches thick;
two from 10 to 12 feet high, and from 2 to 3 inches thick, fastened, at the upper end, to a limb of a tree.

11. A *ladder*, from 12 to 15 feet high; from the top of one rundle to the next a distance of 10 inches.

V. *Estimate of the apparatus of a gymnasium for* 400 *pupils.*

In mentioning the estimate of a gymnastick apparatus, we do not mean to speak of the expense to be incurred in erecting a gymnasium. This would be an useless endeavor, since the expense, resulting from the erecting a gymnasium, depends upon the price of the materials and wages, both of which are different at different times and in different places. Only the quantity of wood and other materials will be given, together with the measures of the single instruments in all their parts.

If a gymnasium is to be erected at the public expense, the cost will form a trifling consideration, if every thing is managed well; if an individual, with limited means, enters upon such an undertaking, he will lessen the expense in a considerable proportion by contracting the climbing-apparatus.

a. Apparatus for leaping.

Two stands for leaping without poles, 6 feet above, 2 feet under ground (4 feet plus 8 feet) equal to 32 feet of wood, from 3 to 4 inches square.

Three stands for leaping with poles, 10 feet above, 3 feet under ground, (6 feet plus 13 feet) equal to 78 feet of wood of 4 inches square. From 20 to 30 feet of wood of the same thickness for steps.

Five pair of iron pegs or bolts, 6 inches long, 1-2 of an inch thick.

Two strings, 10 feet long, 1-2 of an inch thick.

Three strings, 12 feet long, 1-2 of an inch thick.

Ten bags, of any coarse material, filled with sand.

Sixty poles, from 7 to 11 feet long, twelve of each kind.

A ditch for leaping.

Steps for leaping, 24 feet long, resting on four posts, rising from 4 to 10 feet.

b. Vaulting-bars.

1. With saddle-holds.

One 3 feet high; neck 1 foot 10 inches, saddle 1 foot 4 inches, croup 1 foot 6 inches long; the whole length 4 feet 8 inches.

Two 3 feet 4 inches high; neck 2 feet 1 inch, saddle 1

foot 6 inches, croup 1 foot 9 inches long; the whole length 5 feet 4 inches.

Two 3 feet 8 inches high; the other proportions the same as the preceding.

Two 4 feet high; neck 2 feet 4 inches, saddle 1 foot 8 inches, croup 2 feet; the whole length 6 feet.

One 4 feet 4 inches high.

One 4 feet 8 inches high; both of the same length and proportions as the two 4 feet high.

2. Without saddle-holds.

One 3 feet 6 inches high, 4 feet 8 inches long.

One 4 feet high, 5 feet 4 inches long.

One 4 feet 6 inches high, 6 feet long.

The thickness of all is not more than 18, nor less than 14 inches.

This requires two pieces of wood of the trunk of a tree, one 36 feet long, 14 inches thick; the other 30 feet long, 18 inches thick.

For the legs, which are inserted in the trunk about 6 inches, and are as long under, as above ground:

4 (3 feet 6 inches plus 3 feet) equal to 26 feet.

8 (3 feet 10 inches plus 3 feet 4 inches) equal to 57 feet 4 inches.

8 (4 feet 2 inches plus 3 feet 8 inches) equal to 62 feet 8 inches.

8 (4 feet 6 inches plus 4 feet) equal to 68 feet.

4 (4 feet 10 inches plus 4 feet 4 inches) equal to 36 feet 8 inches.

4 (5 feet 2 inches plus 4 feet 8 inches) equal to 48 feet 4 inches.

4 (4 feet plus 3 feet 6 inches) equal to 30 feet.

4 (4 feet 6 inches plus 4 feet) equal to 34 feet.

4 (5 feet plus 4 feet 6 inches) equal to 38 feet.

401 feet of wood are required. The part above ground is wrought to the shape of 4 inches square, the part under ground, unwrought, 6 inches thick, or more.

c. Apparatus for balancing.

Three balancing poles: three masts from 40 to 80 feet long, and at least 12 inches thick at the large end.

For posts:

4 posts 6 feet above ground, 3 feet in ground, equal to 36 feet.

4 posts 4 feet above ground, 3 feet in ground, equal to 28 feet of wood, all of which is 6 inches square.

Four iron bolts, or pegs, upon which two of the masts rest, 2 feet 6 inches long, 1 1-2 inches thick.

The holes bored through the posts, are 6 inches distant from one another.

d. Single bars.

Twelve single bars of eight different heights, each 16 feet long, and resting on three posts:

two 3 feet 6 inches,
two 4 feet,
two 4 feet 6 inches,
two 5 feet,
one 5 feet 6 inches,
one 6 feet,
one 6 feet 6 inches,
one 7 feet above ground.

Twelve poles 16 feet long, 2 1-2 inches thick.

For posts, therefore, which are from 3 feet 6 inches to 7 feet above, and from 2 feet to 3 feet 6 inches under ground:

6 (3 feet 6 inches plus 2 feet) equal to 33 feet,
6 (4 feet plus 2 feet) equal to 36 feet,
6 (4 feet 6 inches plus 2 feet 6 inches) equal to 42 feet,
6 (5 feet plus 2 feet 6 inches) equal to 45 feet,
3 (5 feet 6 inches plus 3 feet) equal to 25 feet 6 inches,
3 (6 feet plus 3 feet) equal to 27 feet,
3 (6 feet 6 inches plus 3 feet 6 inches) equal to 30 feet.
3 (7 feet plus 3 feet 6 inches) equal to 31 feet 6 inches.

270 feet of wood, 5 inches square, are required.

FOUNDATION AND ARRANGEMENT OF A GYMNASIUM. 177

e. Instrument for moving in hanging.

Six poles 9 feet long, 2 1-2 inches thick.

Six posts, 7 feet above, 2 feet under ground, equal to 54 feet of wood, 5 inches square.

f. Parallel bars.

Nine parallel bars, each 10 feet long.

For the upper-pieces, therefore,

18 times 10 feet equal to 180 feet of wood, 3 inches square.

Each bar rests on 4 posts of different height.

One, 2 feet 6 inches above, 1 foot 6 inches in ground, the two parts 1 foot distant.

Two, 3 feet above, 2 feet in ground, the two parts 1 foot 2 inches distant.

Two, 3 feet 6 inches above, 2 feet in ground, the two parts 1 foot 4 inches distant.

Two, 4 feet above, 2 feet in ground, the two parts 1 foot 5 inches distant.

One, 4 feet 6 inches above, 2 feet 6 inches in ground, the two parts 1 foot 6 inches distant.

One, 5 feet above, 2 feet 6 inches in ground, the two parts 1 foot 8 inches distant.

This requires for posts:

4 times 4 feet equal to 16 feet;
8 times 5 feet equal to 40 feet;
8 times 5 feet 6 inches equal to 44 feet;
8 times 6 feet equal to 48 feet;
4 times 7 feet equal to 28 feet;
4 times 7 feet 6 inches equal to 30 feet;
206 feet of wood 4 inches square.

g. Apparatus for climbing.

1. *Ropes*, all of which from 1 1-4 inches to 1 1-2 inches thick, with a firm noose:

two 20 feet long equal to 40 feet,
four 30 feet long equal to 120 feet,
one 40 feet long equal to 40 feet.

In the whole 200 feet.

One rope-ladder, 20 feet long.

2. *Wood.*

For the *instrument with two masts:*

two masts, from 10 to 12 inches thick, 20 feet above, 4 feet in the ground;

two climbing-poles, 3 inches thick, 20 feet above, from 2 to 4 feet in the ground;

two slanting poles, from 4 to 6 inches thick, 24 feet above, 4 feet in the ground;

one beam, from 5 to 6 inches thick, 28 feet long;

two ladders, 24 feet long.

For the *instrument with four masts:*

one mast, from 14 to 18 inches thick, 30 feet above, 6 feet in the ground;

four masts, from 8 to 10 inches thick, 30 feet above, 4 feet in the ground;

four yards, or beams, 6 inches thick, 12 feet long;

one ladder, 35 feet long.

For the *instrument with one mast:*

one mast of considerable thickness, 40 feet above, 8 feet in the ground;

three slanting poles, if possible reaching to the first partition;

for necessary props from 80 to 90 feet of wood;

two boards, 24 feet long;

one ladder, 9 feet long;

one ladder, 16 feet long;

one ladder, 30 feet long.

For the *instrument for climbing by means of the arms alone:*

80 feet of wood, 6 inches square, for the posts and cross-pieces;

20 feet of wood, 4 inches square, for the corner-posts of the upper frame;

130 feet of wood, 3 inches square, for rundles.

Three *climbing-masts*, from 20 to 60 feet, with a cross of oak-wood, fastened below to the mast, by two braces.

 h. Throwing with darts.

For the aim 8 feet of round wood, 6 inches thick;
 a cramp-iron with two strong iron rings.
Twenty darts 6 feet long, 1 1-4 inches thick.
Twenty, 7 feet long, 1 1-4 inches thick.
Twenty, 8 feet long, 1 1-2 inches thick.

 i. Throwing with balls, first kind.

Balls.
 Twelve, of 3 pounds.
 Twelve, of 2 pounds.
 Twelve, of 1 1-2 pounds.
Frame.
 26 feet of wood, 4 inches square.
Planks to cover the first mound.

 j. Throwing with balls, second kind.

A number of balls from 6 to 24 pounds.
A piece of round wood, 8 feet long, from 6 to 8 inches thick.

 k. Drawing.

On one rope from 15 to 20 feet long, 1 inch thick.
On one rope from 30 to 100 feet long, 1 1-2 inches thick.
For two pieces of the instrument for drawing with the neck:
 four girths, from 2 to 3 feet long, from 2 to 3 inches broad, with nooses at both ends;
 four ropes, 10 feet long, 3-4 of an inch thick.
Several staves from 2 to 3 feet long, from 1 1-4 to 1 1-2 inches thick.

 l. Skipping.

Two long ropes from 16 to 20 feet long, 1-2 of an inch thick.

Forty short ropes from 6 to 8 feet long, 1-2 of an inch thick.

Sharp corners and edges, are to be carefully avoided in all kinds of instruments.

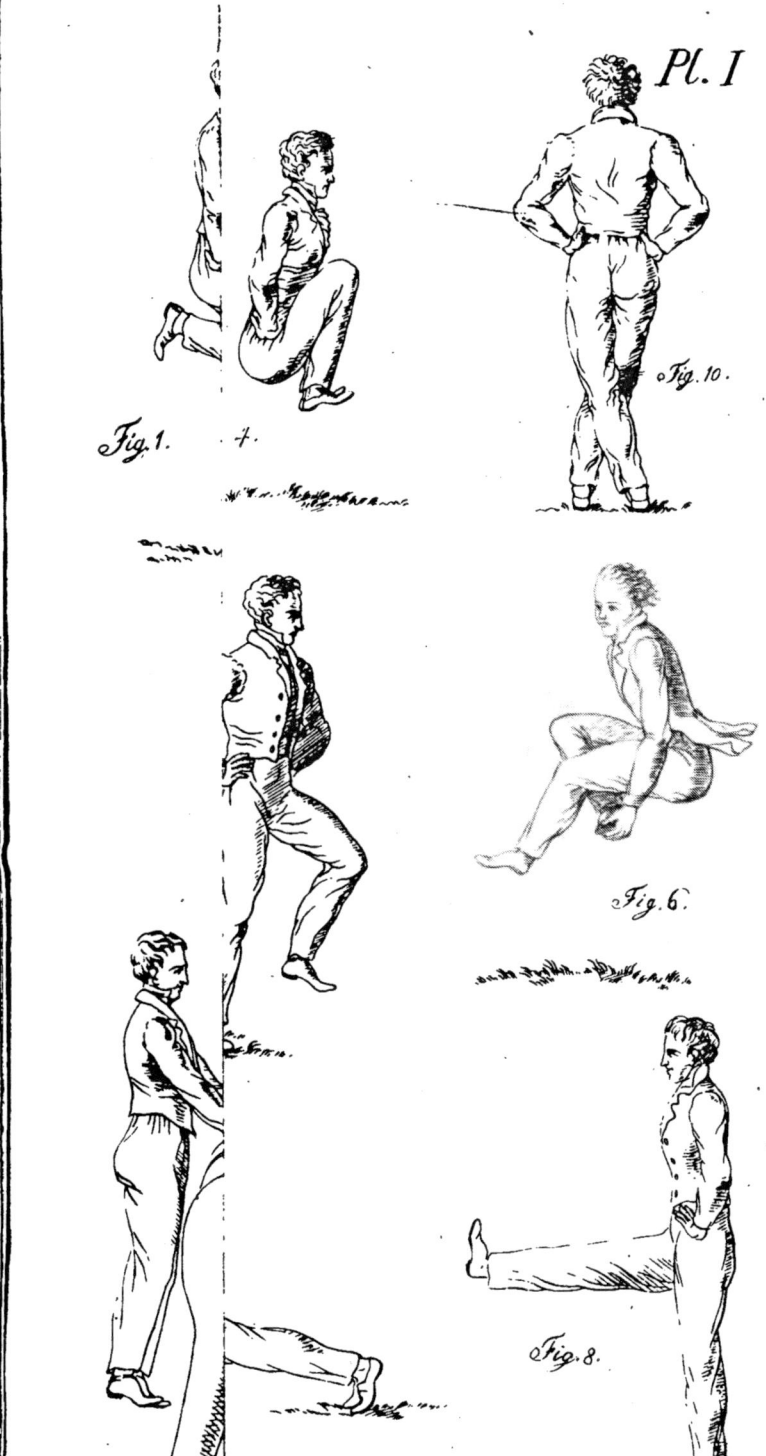

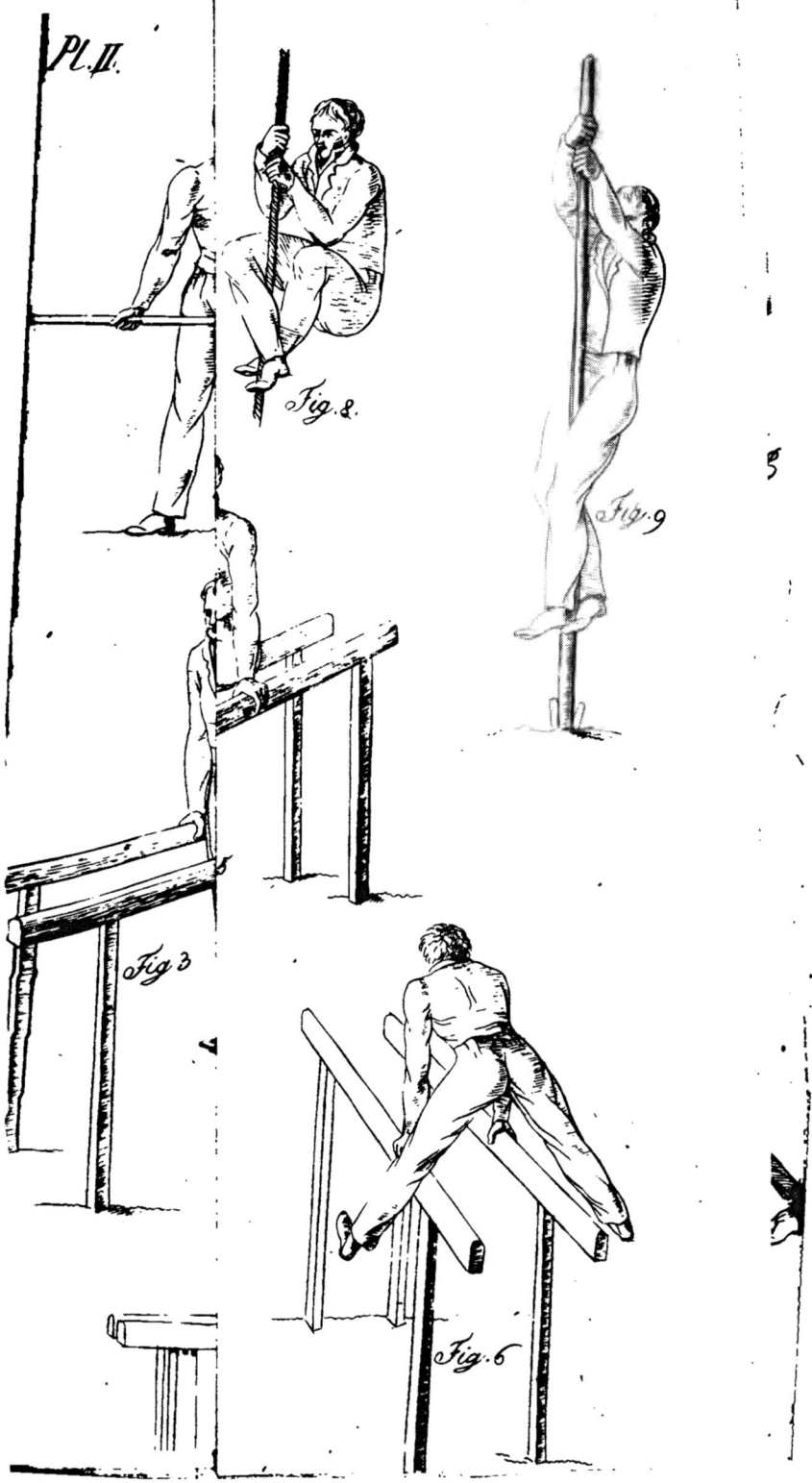

Pl. III

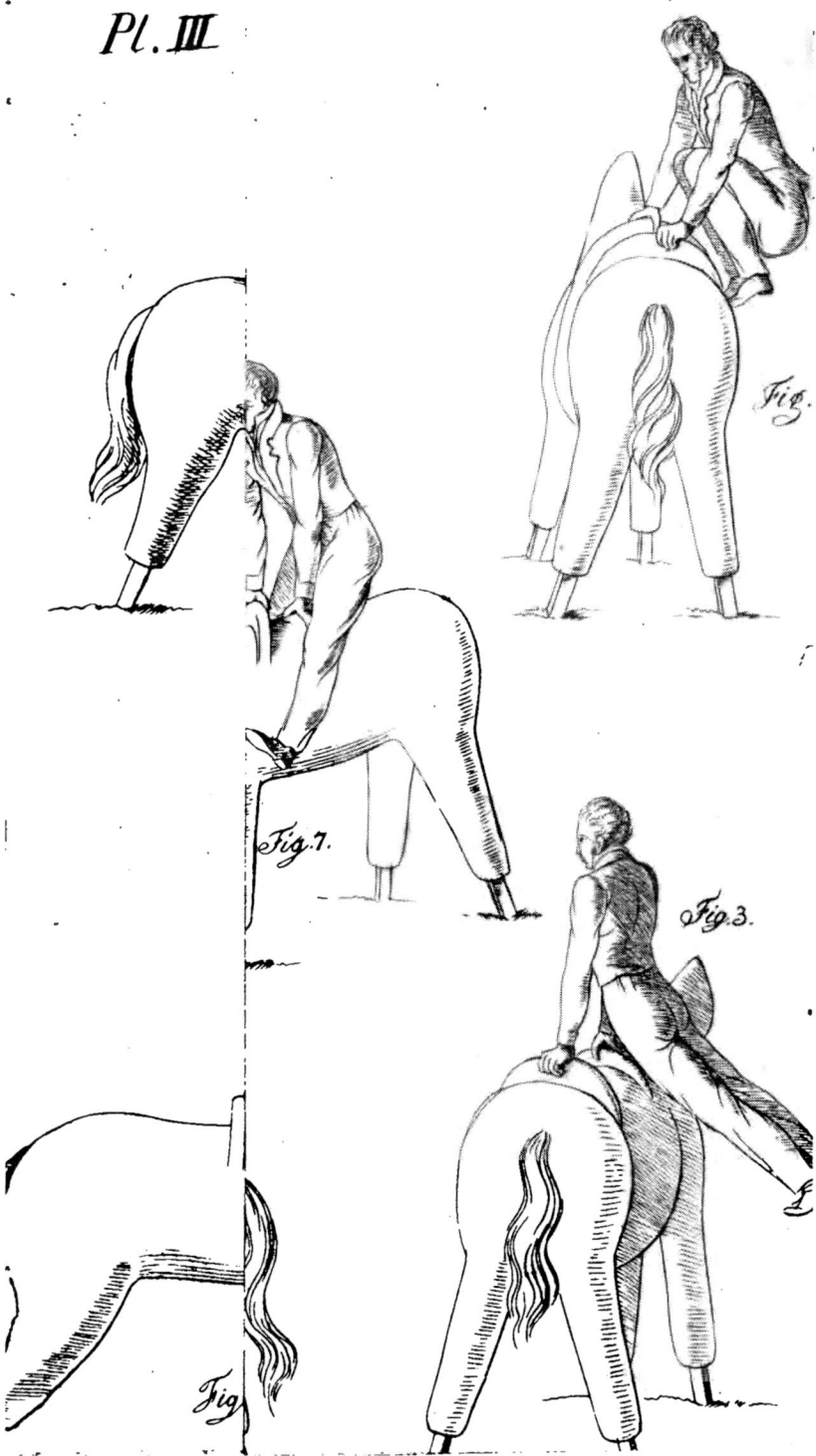

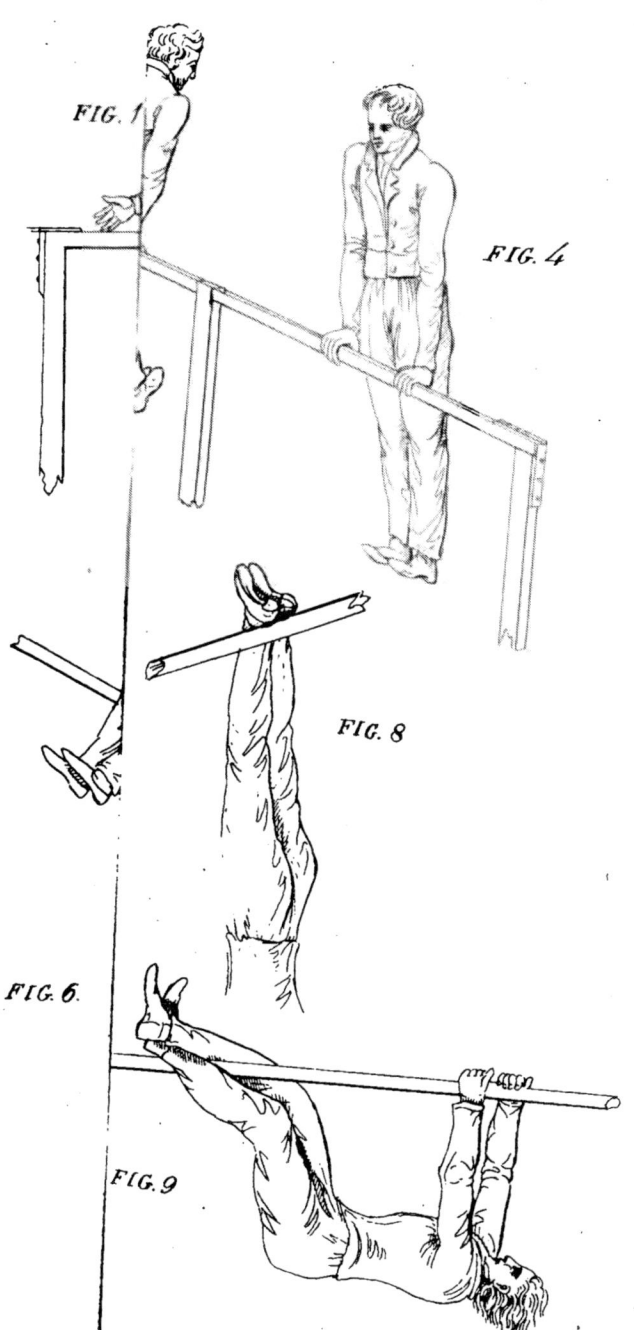

Pl. 4.

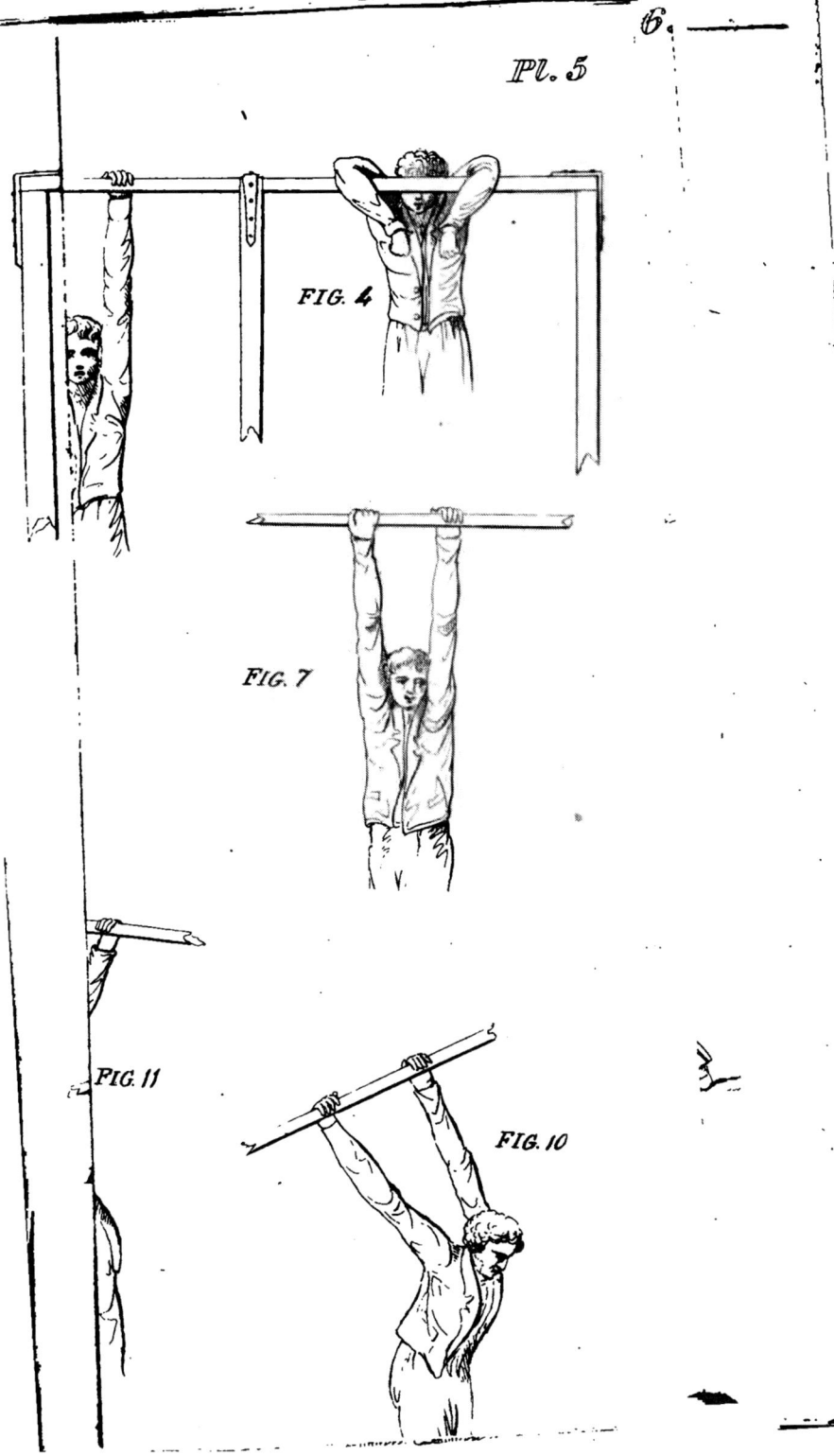

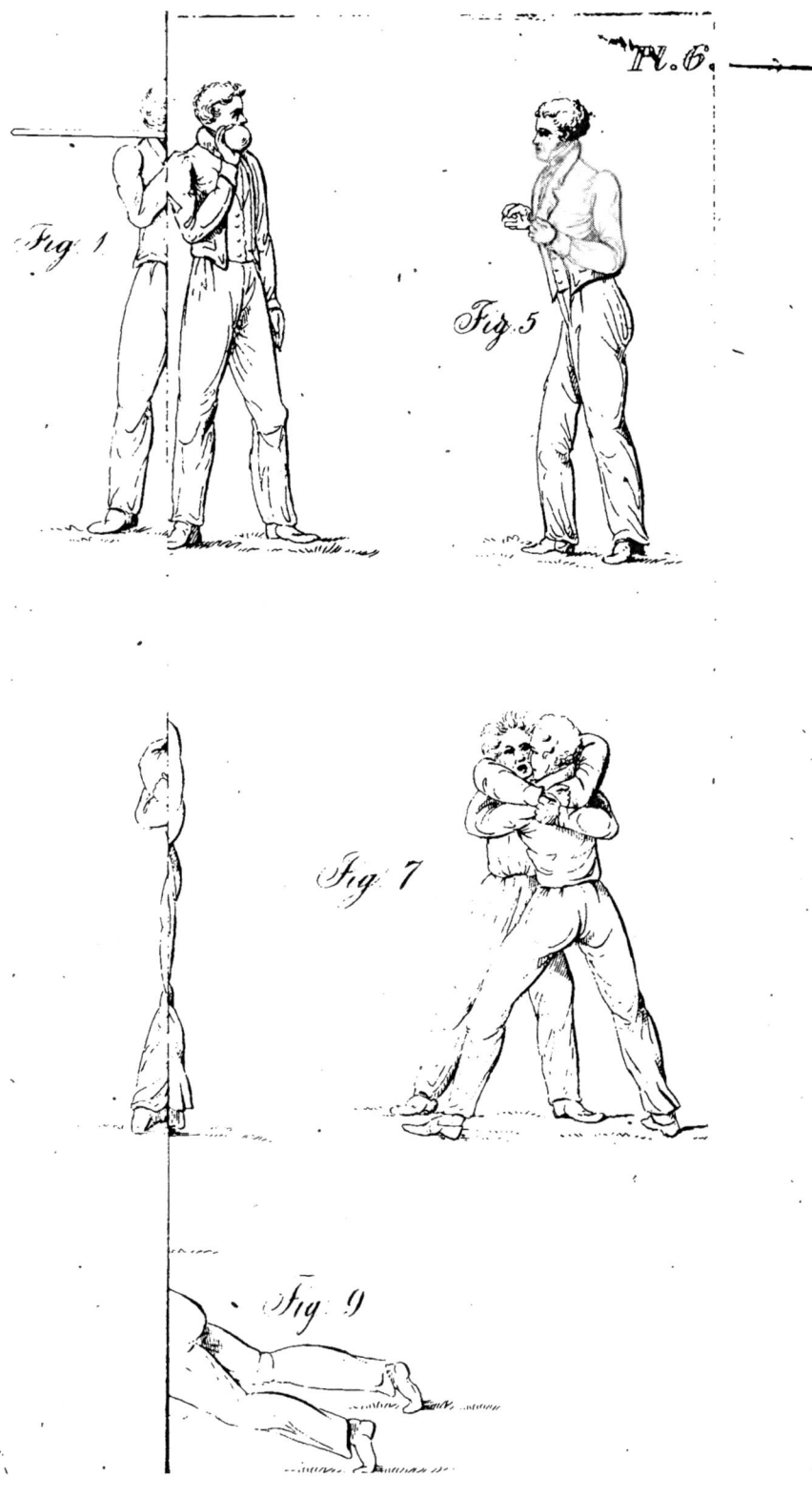

CPSIA information can be obtained at www.ICGtesting.com
Printed in the USA
BVOW03s0638040913

330262BV00012B/400/P